Geriatric
PHARMACOLOGY

The Principles of Practice &
Clinical Recommendations

D1564851

Steven Atkinson, PA-C, MS
Geriatric Internal Medicine

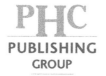

PHC
PUBLISHING
GROUP

*PHC Publishing Group
is an imprint of:*

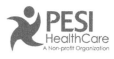

*Continuing Education
Provider since 1979*

2012 Eau Claire, Wisconsin

For information on this book and other continuing education
materials from **PHC Publishing Group** or **PESI HealthCare**
please call **800-843-7763**
or visit our websites
www.phcpublishing.com
www.pesihealthcare.com

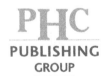

PHC Publishing Group
is an imprint of:

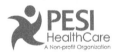

Continuing Education
Provider since 1979

Cover Design: Heidi Knower

Preface

Old age is a time in life where wisdom prevails, but so too does the burden of chronic disease. If only old age didn't require medications to treat and control the symptoms associated with those chronic diseases. And, if only health professionals firmly understood the dynamics of how medications can help, but at the same time hurt, an older adult.

This book was written as a guide for those who seek to provide optimal pharmacotherapy to the geriatric adult. To help those professionals understand what it means to prescribe, dispense and administer medications, but most importantly, manage a combination of those medications safely without causing harm. To help them understand that geriatric adults are more than just "older adults." To prudently look at the changes of aging with a keen eye and the one goal of helping the geriatric adult get the best use of their medications with the least risk.

Moreover, this book is really a compilation of those whom I have centered myself around. People who are brighter and more intellectual, but whose voices I've listened to along the way to create the pages that follow. Here are some of the most influential.

Mom and Dad
Thank you for teaching me that with hard work, sacrifice and self-determination, anything was attainable.

Professor Les Chatelain
For being not only my best mentor but THE ONE who constructively taught me how to educate and to do so with a unique style that captures those I instruct.

(Continued)

Dr. Don Murphy
Despite all your knowledge, for being the humble person who taught me that connecting with a patient is as valuable, if not more valuable, than what a practitioner may actually know.

Dr. Clemenica Rasquinha
For holding my hand along the way, letting go when needed and, most importantly, helping me understand the true art of Geriatric medicine.

Mike Lockwood, PA
For being my most influential teacher in medicine and opening my heart to the world of Geriatrics.

Ellen Balkema, PharmD
For both heightening my interest in, and helping me understand, the critical aspects of geriatric pharmacology.

Dr Greg Gahm (Medical Director)
For helping me critically think, supporting my decisions with the use of evidence, and being a great colleague whom I could always turn to no matter what the circumstance.

About the Author

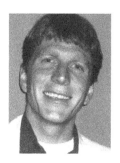

Steven Atkinson, PA-C, MS
Geriatric Internal Medicine

Steven Atkinson is a Board Certified Physician Assistant specializing in Geriatric Internal Medicine. He has been an educator at the University of Utah since 1994 and has been involved in medicine for nearly 22 years. He has been involved in Geriatric Internal Medicine for the last decade and is frequently asked to medically manage the most difficult patients with dementia-related behaviors, those with medication-related problems or those requiring medication adjustments in order to achieve the benefits of therapy. He has published and spoken nationally on dementia and related topics for various audiences. He has also been graciously recognized for his compassionate and dedicated service in Geriatric Medicine by those communities he serves.

Table of Contents

Introduction

Prescribing for the older adult presents unique challenges, yet optimizing drug therapy is an essential part of caring for an older person. In the United States, a Baby Boomer turns sixty every 8 seconds, and by 2030, 20 percent of the United States population is expected to be greater than or equal to 65 years of age (Figure 1-1). In this century, the growth rate of the elderly population has greatly exceeded the growth rate of the country's population as a whole, increasing by a factor of 11 in comparison to that of the previous century.[1] In fact, the oldest old (persons 85 and older) are projected to be the fastest growing part of the elderly population in the coming years.[1]

To combat the health concerns of the aged, medications have become the predominant form of health intervention

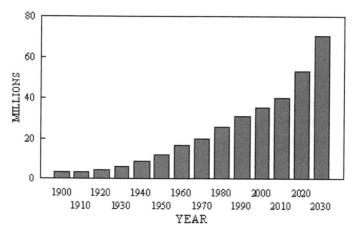

Figure 1-1. Growth of the Elderly Population (1900 - 2030)
Source: Reprinted by permission from U.S. Bureau of Census

today. But as older adults age, there is a strong likelihood for medication errors, adverse drug reactions (ADRs), and adverse drug events (ADEs). It is so significant that nearly 30 percent of all geriatric hospitalizations are the result of an adverse drug event.[2]

The process of prescribing a medication is complex, but the most important question a practitioner should ask when considering a drug is whether the drug is necessary. From that point forward, practitioners need to ensure that they choose the best drug at a dose and schedule appropriate for the patient's physiologic status. They must also monitor for both efficacy and toxicity, educate the patient about desired effects and potential side effects, and consider when that drug may be discontinued.

Geriatric adults carry with them numerous co-morbidities; consequently, they are often prescribed multiple medications for these problems. Medication use increases dramatically with age, with more than 75 percent of Americans older than 60 using two or more prescriptions, and 37 percent using five or more prescriptions.[3] Consequently the risk of an adverse drug event (ADE) is as universal as the drugs that older patients are prescribed.

In weighing the risks and benefits of any medications, practitioners should follow the two mantras of geriatric internal medicine: First, do no harm. Second, start low and go slow. As it applies to risk, the mantras exist because age-related changes in physiology and body habitus compound upon problems that occur in geriatric adults. Since there is such great heterogeneity in the health and functional capacity of older adults, prescribing decisions in this population are more complex and challenging than in any other group of patients in internal medicine. Unlike pediatrics, which for some time has been widely accepted as a distinct entity, geriatrics has yet to achieve this same distinction; therefore, incidence of adverse drug events have been heightened by inappropriate prescribing.

Evidence suggests that inappropriate prescribing is highly prevalent in older people and is associated with an increased risk of ADEs, increased morbidity and mortality, and a growing need for healthcare. These increases occur due to the medical community's failure to identify older adults as distinct individuals who bring to the table distinct co-factors that increase their risk of drug-drug and drug-disease interactions. With the changing demographics and aging population, inappropriate prescribing in older adults should be considered a global healthcare concern.

Currently, elderly adults use approximately 45 percent of the prescription medications that are written.[3] This number is only expected to increase as our population ages and lives longer. But it begs the more important question, WHY?

The answer, "scripts" are driven into our medical system by both patients and physicians, with over 70 percent of all initial consultations resulting in a prescription.[4] In the minds of a practitioner and a patient, a prescription often signifies the end of a consultation; it means something has been done. But the misunderstanding in geriatrics is that advice can be as powerful a tool as a prescription itself. Certainly, there are those patients who describe themselves as being cheated when scripts aren't written, and consequently, prescribers reluctantly give in to their demands. But for the most part, older adults find comfort in their geriatric provider, and if that provider takes time to explain why a drug is not being chosen, the patient often is willing to wait.

Why does the trend of "pill-pushing" pose such a significant risk in geriatrics? First and foremost, no studies can predict the consequences of multiple, simultaneous medications in any population, let alone one that is already frail and at higher risk of an adverse drug event. Instead, practitioners rely on their experience, instincts, and education about "a" drug to make decisions about an array of drugs. Unfortunately, even the most well trained practitioners have difficulty predicting drug-drug interactions (DDIs). Second, physiological changes make the elderly more sensitive to medications. Finally, drug-disease interactions tend to be more common in older adults. In order to improve health outcomes, providers need to find a balance between prescribing medically necessary and safe medications and preventing adverse drug events. My hope is that this book will teach readers how to do that.

To qualify this more distinctly: *It is possible to arrive at a group of medications that has clear relevance to care, that is scientifically valid, usable, and feasible, and that doesn't place the patient at a significant risk!*

Chapter 1
Pathophysiological Principles of Aging

Pharmacokinetics, or what the body does to a drug, is affected by four factors in any patient: absorption, distribution, metabolism and elimination (ADME). However, an older adult's unique and important physiological changes affect the rate by which drugs are absorbed, distributed, metabolized, or eliminated in the body. Ultimately, these changes synergistically affect the levels of drugs in the blood stream to potentiate drug toxicity.

Since metabolism and excretion of drugs decrease in the elderly, toxicity may develop slowly and sometimes go unrecognized. As a general rule, drugs don't reach steady-state until about five half-lives of the drug in question. Steady-state is the level at which a drug rises in the body (blood and tissue) until it plateaus and is essentially at the same level in the body at all times.

Since it takes five of these half-lives to plateau, toxic effects of medications may be delayed, especially if the half-life is long. As an example, the benzodiazepines diazepam (Valium') has a half-life up to nearly 96 hours in many elderly patients. Since it takes five half-lives before a drug reaches steady-state, signs of toxicity may not appear until 20 days after initial and subsequent ingestion. The equation below elaborates on this.

96 hours × 5 half-lives/24 hours = 20 days until steady-state

In the arena of pharmacokinetics, there are four factors that influence the possibility of either toxicity or drug interaction.

Absorption

Absorption is the process of a substance entering the blood circulation. Once inside the body, the medication is then described by how available it is to that organism. As people age, absorption rates fluctuate. Some physiological alterations that affect absorption include a decrease in gastric secretion, an increase in gastric pH, a decrease in gastrointestinal blood flow and motility, and a decrease in pancreatic trypsin. But of the four pharmacokinetic processes, absorption has the least significant impact on the elderly patient.

Non-physiological factors, on the other hand, *do affect* absorption. Many older adults take supplements such as multivitamins, calcium, magnesium, and iron, all of which can affect the absorption of other prescription medications taken with it. For example, if a patient takes phenytoin (Dilantin˚) with calcium, absorption is affected in such a way that it may decrease serum phenytoin levels. If oral levofloxacin (Levaquin˚) is given with oral iron (ferrous sulfate or ferrous gluconate), it affects the absorption of levofloxacin and decreases the availability of the antibiotic. That is, it affects how well the antibiotic works.

Although this is not a given rule, it is a general one: separate supplements of any kind from active medications by at least two hours in any direction.

Distribution

Unlike absorption, drug distribution changes with age because of physiological changes in body composition in the elderly. *Distribution* is the dispersion or dissemination of substances throughout the fluids and tissues of the body. Those physiological changes include a decrease, by up to 20 percent of lean body weight and total body water, an increase in body fat by up to 35 percent, and an 8-10 percent decrease in serum albumin, a means by which many drugs are transported through the body.

Increased fat can affect the volume of distribution (Vd) for highly lipophilic drugs and consequently may decrease the elimination of that drug leading to toxicity. It has long been shown that medications used in surgical anesthesia have an effect in older patients that is related to this physiological increase in body fat. Vecuronium (Norcuron˚), pancuronium

(Pavulon˙), and morphine are some common examples.[5] This effect explains why it is not uncommon to see delirium long after surgery in older adults. The implications of this in older adults is serious, since drugs that affect the Central Nervous System (CNS) are then delayed in their ability to leave the body.

Decreased body water affects hydrophilic drugs such as digoxin and lithium. With a decrease in body water there is also a decrease in the Vd of hydrophilic drugs. In relationship to lithium, it means there is less circulating lithium available to that individual.

Practically speaking, this means that in an older adult, hydrophilic drugs reach steady-state more quickly and are eliminated more expeditiously compared with lipophilic medications that require more time to reach steady-state but are also eliminated at a slower rate.[6]

As lean body weight is reduced, there is also a reduction in serum albumin. This reduction may enhance the drug effects because serum levels of an unbound drug may increase. For example, the fraction of unbound phenytoin (Dilantin˙) has been shown to increase 25 to 40 percent in older patients as a consequence of this principle. This same principle explains why warfarin (Coumadin˙) is harder to regulate in patients with reduced lean body weight.

In addition, drugs are distributed to different places in the body depending on their chemical structure. Those changes affect the amount of drug needed to produce a desired therapeutic outcome. Inappropriately adjusted medications can lead to toxicity or undesired side effects in the elderly.

The most significant example of this effect is the drug digoxin. Used commonly in heart disease, this drug distributes to the muscle. In a geriatric adult, since lean body mass is reduced and digoxin itself has a very narrow therapeutic range, toxicity may occur and is likely, since this drug is less able to bind to muscle. But there are other examples as well: antibiotics, carbamazepine, lithium, benzodiazepines, and theophylline are all affected by this principle.

Metabolism

Metabolism describes how a drug is converted from its parent compound into its daughter metabolites. These alternate compounds may be pharmacologically active or inactive. In general, overall hepatic metabolism of many drugs through the cytochrome P-450 enzyme system decreases with age. For those drugs with decreased hepatic metabolism, clearance would be reduced, and theoretically is reduced, by approximately 30 to 40 percent. This effect would indicate that maintenance drug doses in the elderly should be decreased by this percentage; however, rate of drug metabolism varies greatly from person to person, and individual titration is required.

Elimination

Elimination is the process of removing compounds from the body. It is a true measure of how a drug is removed from the body expressed as volume per unit of time. Drug elimination in older adults is also reduced because of the reductions in renal blood flow, kidney size, and glomerular filtration that accompany both physiological changes and age-related chronic conditions.

Half Life ($t_{1/2}$)

Another concept important in elimination of drugs is known as half-life ($t_{1/2}$). *Half-life* is the amount of time for a drug to decline by 50 percent in the serum. It can be expressed in seconds, minutes, hours, or even days. For example, the cardiac medication adenosine (Adenocard') has a half-life of less than 10 seconds. On the other hand, the cardiac medication amiodorone (Pacerone') has a half-life of approximately 58 days. Drug handbooks usually have detailed accounts of the half-life of any medication. Pharmacists are also a handy resource when this information is needed.

Medications can have one of several fates. They can be eliminated from the body (as discussed earlier), or they can be moved to another body fluid compartment such as the intracellular fluid; they can also be destroyed in the blood. The removal of a drug from the plasma is known as *clearance,* and the distribution of the drug into the various body tissues is known as the *volume of distribution.* Both of these pharmacokinetic parameters are important in determining the half-life of a drug and also represent the transition to another important concept in geriatric pharmacology: pharmacodynamics.

But since metabolism and excretion decrease as adults age, toxicity may develop slowly because medications take around five days to reach steady-state. The earlier example that was given to discuss this was diazepam (Valium®). A significant additional example includes chlordiazepoxide (Librium®). This medication has active metabolites with half-lives up to 200 hours in some cases. Consequently, a practitioner may not see the side effects for up to 1000 hours after the medication is initiated.

200 hours × 5 half-lives = 1000 hours

Chapter 2
Understanding Renal Elimination in Older Adults

After age 30, creatinine clearance (CrCl) begins to decrease by an average of 8 mL/min/1.73 m²/decade (Figure 2-1).

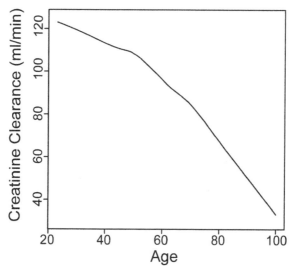

Figure 2-1. Approximate Age Related Decline Creatinine Clearance

However, there is a great degree of variability when it comes to the age-related decrease in renal function. Consequently, using estimated creatinine clearance (Figure 2-2) can result in erroneous calculations about how well the kidney is actually functioning in an older adult. This variation occurs because muscle mass is reduced in older adults; therefore, less creatinine is also produced. By using standard equations that measure CrCl, such as Cockcroft-Gault, true kidney function can be underestimated, and drug toxicity could result.

$$CrCl = \frac{(140 - age) \bullet Wt}{S_{Cr} \bullet 72}(\bullet 0.85)$$

Women only

Figure 2-2. Estimated Creatinine Clearance (CrCl)

Better indicators of kidney function in older adults include an estimated glomerular filtration rate (Figure 2-3) since decreases in tubular function parallel those seen in glomerular function. Nephrologists, as specialists in the kidney, nearly always speak in terms of estimated glomerular filtration (eGRF) rates.

This concept is often poorly understood even by the most astute practitioners. To elaborate, to use serum creatinine alone is not an accurate index of the level of eGFR. The National Kidney Foundation asserts that the use of the serum levels of creatinine as an index of GFR rests on three important assumptions: (1) creatinine is an ideal filtration marker whose clearance approximates GFR; (2) creatinine excretion rate is constant among individuals and over time; and (3) measurement of serum creatinine is accurate and reproducible across clinical laboratories.[7] Since these assumptions are not true in the elderly, estimated Glomerular Filtration Rate (eGFR) is the tool that should be used to assess true kidney function

$$GFR^{MDRD/IDMS} = 175 \times S_{cr}^{-1.154} \times Age^{-0.203} \times \begin{array}{l} \text{(0.742 if female)} \\ \text{(1.212 if African American)} \end{array}$$

Figure 2-3. Estimated Glomerular Filtration Rate (eGFR)

The following graph (Figure 2-4) demonstrates the relationship between serum creatinine, creatinine clearance, and glomerular filtration rate.

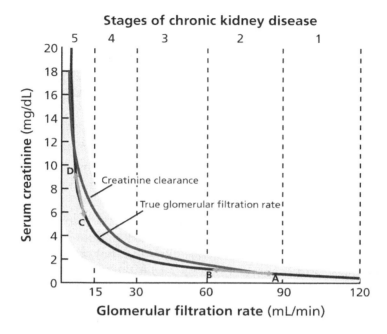

Figure 2-4. Relationship Between Serum Creatinine, CrCl and GFR

Source: Reprinted by permission from Elsevier.

As demonstrated in Figure 2-4, large changes in GFR are reflected by only very small changes in serum creatinine (points A to B). Conversely, minute changes in GFR are reflected by large changes in serum creatinine (points C to D).[8] This phenomenon can cause practitioners to view small changes in creatinine as insignificant, especially in patients with creatinine levels in the normal or near-normal range.

As is noted in Figure 2-4, even small changes in serum creatinine, from roughly 1.0 to 1.8 mg/dL, *can* and *do* represent large changes in GFR (e.g., 88 to 62 mL/min/1.73 m^2). This is one of the main reasons the National Kidney Foundation created equations specific for eGFR. As a general rule, for every doubling of serum creatinine (SCr), creatinine clearance decreases by 50 percent. For example, if SCr changes from 1.0 - 2.0 mg/dl, kidney function is reduced by 50 percent, whereas a change in SCr from, say, 4.0 - 6.0 mg/dl is less significant (approximately a 25 percent reduction) in terms of kidney function.

The best models for estimations in glomerular filtration can be found at:
http://www.kidney.org/professionals/tools/index.cfm

From there, practitioners need only plug in the numbers to get an accurate description of kidney function. Additionally, practitioners can download free applications to smart phones that will allow them to have access to eGFR at any time. These estimates are important when they relate to medication dosing as described by Chronic Kidney Disease. More importantly, they will minimize an adverse drug event when prescribing medications for older adults.

Chronic Kidney Disease (CKD) is the slow loss of kidney function over time, and it occurs in every patient and in every adult. The loss of function usually—but not always—occurs over years, and is best defined based on the eGFR as estimated by the Modification of Diet in Renal Disease (MDRD) equation described earlier.

The definition of CKD was established by the National Kidney Foundation in 2002 and for practical purposes in geriatrics is defined as a persistent eGFR $< 60mL/min/1.73m^2$ on two tests at least three months apart. The definition contains two components—kidney damage and duration. This has significant implications in the elderly since a decreased eGFR is an independent predictor of adverse outcomes, such as cardiovascular disease and *death*. As a better clinical indicator, two independent studies showed that when eGFR was less than 50 $mL/min/1.73m^2$, there was a significant increase in mortality.[9,10] Any eGFR that demonstrates CKD in the elderly requires adjustment in drug dosages for maximizing safety and minimizing mortality.

Chronic Kidney Disease is classified and defined by "levels" or stages (Table 2-1). The stages of CKD are essentially based on measured or estimated Glomerular Filtration Rate. There are five stages, but for practical purposes, kidney function in the elderly is essentially insignificant in Stage 1 and only minimally reduced in Stage 2. As was mentioned earlier, in older adults, Stage III CKD or greater indicates impairment, which *requires* dosing adjustments and consideration of the potential for harm when introducing medications.

14

Table 2-1. Stages of Chronic Kidney Disease

Stage	GFR (mL/min/1.73 m²)	Description
I	≥90	Normal kidney function but structural abnormalities suggest kidney disease
II	60-89	Mildly reduced kidney function
III	30-59	Moderately reduced kidney function
IV	15-29	Severely reduced kidney function
V	<15	End-Stage Renal Disease (ESRD)

Adapted from National Kidney Foundation Kidney Disease Outcomes Quality Initiative (KDOQI) Guidelines (NKF, 2002).

With that understanding, practitioners can now make reasonable considerations about dose adjustments of medications, but more importantly, not overlook the use of serum creatinine alone as a tool to measure overall kidney function. The following (Table 2-2) clearly demonstrates how serum creatinine underestimates glomerular filtration and thereby may lead to risky practicing techniques that could cause harm.

Table 2-2. Comparison of SCr and eGFR

	22 year-old African-American Man	60 year-old Caucasian Man	79 year-old Caucasian Woman
Serum creatinine	1.2mg/dL	1.2mg/dL	1.2 mg/dL
GFR (MDRD equation)	98 mL/min/1.73 m2	65 mL/min/1.73 m2	46 mL/min/1.73 m2
Classification of CKD	Normal GFR	Stage II CKD	Stage III CKD

This table demonstrates the significant degree to which kidney function can be reduced when looking at the whole picture rather than at creatinine alone.

Table 2-3 takes this a step further by comparing creatinine clearance with glomerular filtration rate. It is meant to demonstrate risks associated with using CrCl over what should be considered the gold standard: eGFR.

Table 2-3. Comparison of SCr and eGFR

Age	Serum Cr	Creatinine Clearance	GFR
(years)	(mg/dL)	(mL/min)	(mL/min/1.73 m^2)
30	1.1	64	62
50	1.1	52	56
70	1.1	41	49
85	1.1	32	47

As can clearly be seen in Table 2-3, using CrCl could markedly underestimate how the kidney is actually functioning (especially as the patient ages). In the patient used in this example, CrCl remains well preserved even up to 85 years of age. But as a comparison, eGFR is at stage III CKD as early as age 50 in this same patient. Even more alarming, by age 70, this patient's eGFR suggests an increased risk of death despite a CrCl that is fairly well preserved.[9,10]

Chapter 3
Aging and Pharmacodynamics

Pharmacodynamics is the study of the biochemical and physiological effects of drugs on the body. Pharmacodynamics, along with pharmacokinetics (what the body does to a drug), explains the mechanisms of drug action and the relationship between drug concentration and an individual's response to that drug. In older adults, the effects of similar drug concentrations (sensitivity) may be greater or smaller than those in younger people. As an example, older adults receiving morphine sulfate are more prone to an acute analgesic effect. That is, they are more prone to sedation with the same dose of morphine sulfate than are younger adults. Albuterol, on the other hand, has a less potent effect on older adults than it does on younger adults. As a general rule, expect sensitivities to most drugs to be enhanced or heightened in the elderly.

Some common drug categories posing risks to older adults include analgesics, anticoagulants, antihypertensives, antiparkinsonian drugs, diuretics, hypoglycemic drugs, and psychoactive drugs, to name a few. But in general, pharmacodynamics is of particular importance when medicines like these are prescribed since they pose a risk of falls and fractures and can be lethal for older adults. This is explained in more detail in Chapters 4-7.

Optimal pharmacotherapy in the elderly is a delicate balance between overprescribing and under-prescribing. Realistically, it is a balance between choosing the correct drug, at the correct dose, that targets the appropriate condition. But it is MOST important to ask if the drug is necessary for the patient. The word "necessary" should really be a practitioner's reflection on considering non-pharmacological approaches to treatment first, then considering whether a pharmacological approach is indeed necessary. An unknown but highly intellectual source is quoted as saying: *avoid a pill for every ill.*

Table 3-1 lists inappropriate or overprescribed medications; however, just as there are those medications that are inappropriately prescribed, there are, as well, those medications that tend to be under-prescribed.

Table 3-1. Common Inappropriate/Overprescribed and Under-prescribed Medications/Classes[11]

Inappropriate / Overprescribed
anticholinergic agents
urinary and GI antispasmodics
antipsychotics
benzodiazepines
digoxin for diastolic dysfunction
dipyridamole
H2-receptor antagonists
laxatives and fecal softeners
NSAIDs (non-steroidal anti-inflammatory drugs)
PPIs (proton-pump inhibitors)
sedating antihistamines (H1-receptor antagonists, e.g., diphenhydramine)
TCAs (triclyclic antidepressants)
vitamins and minerals

Under-prescribed
ACE inhibitors for patients with diabetes and proteinuria
ARBs (angiotensin-receptor blockers)
anticoagulants
antihypertensive and diuretics as evidenced by uncontrolled hypertension
B-blockers for patients after MI or with heart failure
bronchodilators
PPIs or misoprostol for GI protection when taking NSAIDs
statins (until certain comorbidities are reached)
vitamin D and calcium for patients with or at risk of osteoporosis

Adapted from: Pacala JT, Sullivan GM, eds. *American Geriatrics Society*; 2010.

It is important to remember that this list should serve as a guideline, not a rule. As is noted above, limiting medications to avoid overprescribing can result in under-prescribing. The harm that comes from under-prescribing is as unjust as that of overprescribing.

Under-prescribing usually occurs from practitioners' nihilistic notion that older adults will not benefit from medications intended for primary or secondary prevention, or from aggressive management of chronic conditions like hypertension, diabetes, COPD, osteoporosis or congestive heart failure. In one study, underuse of medications was found to be as high as 64 percent.[12]

On the other hand, the potential consequences of overprescribing include adverse drug events, drug-drug interactions, duplicative therapy, and increased costs. Medicine is called an art because it is a balance of enhancing both quantity and quality of life, but doing so safely.

Chapter 4

Adverse Drug Events

Adverse drug events (ADEs) are any injury resulting from drug therapy. They are the most serious consequence of inappropriate prescribing. Common ADEs are over-sedation, falls and fractures, bleeding, hallucinations, and confusion. More than 95 percent of ADEs that occur in the elderly are considered predictable, and approximately 50 percent are considered preventable.[13] In the United States over two million serious adverse drug events (ADEs) occur annually and account for over 100,00 deaths. If ADEs were ranked as a disease, it would be between the fourth and sixth leading cause of death in the United States.[14,15]

Although adverse drug effects can occur in any patient, certain characteristics of the elderly make them more susceptible to adverse effects. The elderly, for example, often take many more drugs than their younger counterparts. Consequently, this "polypharmacy" adds to risk. Additionally, both age-related changes in physiology (Chapters 1 and 2) and the pharmacodynamics and pharmacokinetics of drugs (Chapter 3) increase the risks of an adverse effect. In fact, the relationship between adverse drug events and the number of drugs is corollary. After 5 PRESCRIBED medications, the percentage of patients with adverse effects nearly doubles. Once 9 prescription medications are breached, there is a 100% risk of an adverse drug event (*see Figure 4-1*).[16]

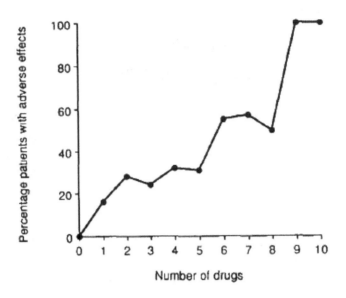

Figure 4-1. Relationship Between Prescription Drug and Adverse Drug Events

The primary reason for ADEs in the elderly is inappropriate prescribing. A drug is inappropriately prescribed if its potential for harm outweighs its potential for benefit. Common examples of inappropriate prescribing include unsuitable drug choices, too high of a dose, dosing that is too frequent, a long duration of therapy, duplicative therapy, failure to consider drug interactions, and incorrect indications for a drug. Drugs that are mistakenly continued once an acute condition resolves (as may happen when patients move from one health care setting to another) is another common example of inappropriate prescribing. In fact, up to 30 percent of hospital admissions in older people are related to adverse drug events that directly relate to inappropriate prescribing. [2]

A number of drug categories (e.g., antihypertensives, analgesics, anticoagulants, diuretics, hypoglycemic drugs, and psychoactive drugs) pose significant risks for elderly patients and will be discussed in greater detail in Chapters 5 and 6.

Beers' Criteria has cited drugs that pose the biggest risk to older adults (*see Chapter 6*). It was initially developed in 1991 by a group of 12 clinicians with expertise in geriatrics and led by Dr. Mark Beers. The "Beers List" has literally dominated the international literature since its development in 1991 and has been updated three times since, with the latest revision in 2012. In retrospect, despite some criticism of its development, Dr. Mark Beers' criteria have served as a dedicated approach to improving administration and safety of drugs in the underserved geriatric adult.

Additionally, the STOPP (Screening Tool of Older Persons' potentially inappropriate Prescriptions) and START (Screening Tool to Alert doctors to the Right Treatment) criteria have been validated as a tool for appropriate prescribing in older adults (*see Chapter 7*). STOPP and START are arranged according to physiological systems and include reference to drug-drug and drug-disease interactions. Unlike Beers, these tools address the domains of prescribing *appropriateness*. Clinicians, however, are still left to weigh these guidelines and to determine the benefits and risks of therapy in each patient, since some patients may actually BENEFIT from drugs listed on the Beers Criteria or on STOPP and START. As has been pointed out, these tools are guidelines to maximize safety and minimize harm.

Despite the Beers Criteria and STOPP and START, inappropriate drugs are still being prescribed for the elderly with little consideration to safety; in one survey, as many of 40 percent of nursing-home residents were using at least one inappropriate drug.[11] In such patients, not only does the risk of hospitalization increase, but the risk of death increases as well.

For older adults in a community-based environment, medication classes most frequently implicated in adverse drug events are listed in Table 4-1.[17]

Table 4-1. Most Frequent Drug Classes Causing ADEs in Community-Dwelling Adults

Most frequent drug class causing ADEs	Percentage (%) of incidence
Cardiovascular active agents	34
Analgesics (opioids/benzo's)	18
Antibiotics	15
Hypoglycemic agents	10
Psychotropic agents	7
Anticoagulants	5
Others (NSAIDS, Anticholinergics)	11

Source: From Professor Graham Davies, Professor of Clinical Pharmacy & Therapeutics. Reprinted with permission.

Of the classes of medications listed above, warfarin (Coumadin®), digoxin (Digitek®, Lanoxin®) and insulin (Humulin®, Novolin®) account for 1/3 of ALL adverse drug events.[18] However, many inappropriate drugs are available over-the-counter (OTC) as well *(see Table 5-9)*. So clinicians should always question patients about the use of OTC drugs and herbal agents in order to have a full understanding of potential drug-drug-interactions as well as adverse drug events that may occur.

In nursing homes, as is shown in Table 4-2, agents causing the most severe adverse drug events vary by only a small degree with that of the community-based group.

Table 4-2. Most Frequent Drug Classes Causing ADEs in Nursing Home Residents

Most frequent drug class causing ADEs in nursing home residents	Percentage (%) of incidence
Cardiovascular active agents	36
Analgesics agents	13
CNS Agents	19
ASA	7

Source: From Professor Graham Davies, Professor of Clinical Pharmacy & Therapeutics. Reprinted with permission.

In general, when older adults are prescribed drugs for minor symptoms, practitioners should consider if a non-pharmacological approach could be considered or be even more appropriate. If practitioners decide that pharmacological treatment is warranted (e.g., analgesics, H2-blockers, hypnotics, or laxatives) then they should consider writing time-limited prescriptions (e.g., Duonebs 4x/day for one week then discontinue.)

Solving the problem of inappropriate prescribing in the elderly is not just about considering a short list of drugs and noting drug categories of concern. Inappropriate prescribing is remedied by a constant review of a patient's entire drug regimen, evaluating benefit and harm, and making sure "new" conditions aren't the result of an adverse drug event. By doing so, practitioners are more likely to avoid overprescribing or the consequence of a "prescribing cascade."

A *prescribing cascade* occurs when the side effect of a drug is misinterpreted as a sign or symptom of a new disorder, leading to a new drug being prescribed to treat that effect. This situation is heightened when the new, unnecessary drug causes additional side effects, which may then be misinterpreted as yet another disorder and treated unnecessarily (Figure 4-2).[19]

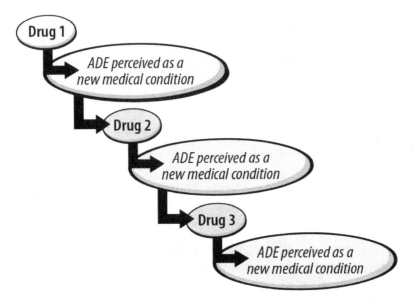

Figure 4-2. The "Prescribing Cascade"

Many drugs have adverse effects that resemble symptoms or disorders common in the elderly. Here are some common examples:

NSAIDs > HTN >> anti-hypertensive therapy initiated

Non-Steroidal Anti-Inflammatory Drugs (NSAIDs) have long been known to cause hypertension (HTN) as well as many other side effects. Patients may become hypertensive (HTN), so anti-hypertensive agents are initiated, and thus a prescribing cascade is born.

NSAIDs > blood in stool >> H2-blocker >>> delirium >>>>Haldol initiated

Non-Steroidal Anti-Inflammatory Drugs (NSAIDs) are the most common medicinal cause of GI bleeding. As a consequence of the GI bleeding, H2-blockers are started. H2-blockers have been known to result in delirium because of their anti-cholinergic properties. The delirium then leads to a very dangerous prescribing cascade: the initiation of haloperidol (Haldol®) to manage the behaviors associated with the delirium.

metoclopramide > Parkinsonism >> carbidopa/levodopa initiated >>> fludrocortisone for hypotension

Metoclopramide (Reglan®) has side effects that mimic Parkinson's disease. Those features can lead to the initiation of carbidopa/levodopa (Sinemet®), which has a side effect of hypotension. The next step in the cascade is the subsequent use of fludrocortisone (Florinef®) to treat the hypotension.

HCTZ > gout >> NSAIDs >>> antihypertensive initiated

A side effect of thiazide diuretics such as hydrochlorothiazide (HCTZ) is an increase in serum uric acid levels, which can consequently lead to the development of gout. The cascade that follows is the use of NSAIDs to treat the gout. Subsequently, the patient may get hypertensive, leading to the initiation of anti-hypertensives.

SSRIs > hyponatremia >> declomycin

The rate of SSRI/SNRI-induced hyponatremia ranges between .5–32%. Consequently, declomycin may have to be initiated to treat the hyponatremia.

OTC pseudoephedrine > urinary retention >> alpha blocker

Over-the-counter (OTC) pseudoephedrine has been associated with urinary retention due to its mechanism of action. Consequently, an alpha-blocker, which incidentally does the exact opposite of pseudoephedrine, may have to be initiated to treat the retention.

antipsychotic > extra pyramidal side-effects >> primidone

The classes of antipsychotic agents are quite large nowadays, but even the newer agents are associated with extrapyramidal side effects (EPS). Should these side effects occur, it is not uncommon to use primidone (Mysoline®) as a treatment option leading to a prescribing cascade.

cholinesterases > urinary incontinence >> oxybutinin

The classes of medications known as cholinesterases usually include cognitive enhancers. A common side effect of the cholinesterases (Aricept®, Razadyne®, Exelon®) is urinary incontinence. Consequently, oxybutinin (Ditropan®) may get initiated to treat the urinary problem.

As a general rule, all practitioners should evaluate ANY new symptom and treat it as an adverse drug event before considering starting a "new" medication to treat it. To evaluate and compare med-lists from 2 months prior is a methodology that practitioners should be accustomed to. In itself, this will help minimize falling victim to the prescribing cascade.

Here are some additional rules to follow to minimize the risk of a prescribing cascade:

- Assume any new symptoms are drug-related until proven otherwise.
- Monitor patients for signs or symptoms of adverse drug effects.
    - measure drug levels where appropriate
    - monitor laboratory tests where appropriate
- Document the expected response to therapy and discontinue or up titrate therapy if this goal is not achieved.
- Document the risk and benefit of any medicinal therapy, but, more importantly, justify whether the drug therapy is medically necessary.

Chapter 5
Drug-Drug Interactions

A *drug-drug interaction* (DDI) is a modification of the effect of a drug when administered with another drug.[20] It is known to increase as the number of medications a patient takes increases, as the age and frailty of the patient increases, as the number of physicians involved in a patient's care increases, and occurs when patients use more than one pharmacy or pharmacy shop. Common adverse events that occur from DDIs include delirium, hypotension, and acute kidney injury.

As was discussed earlier, drug interactions can take many forms. A relatively common and significant site of DDIs involves the cytochrome P-450 (CYP450) system. The CYP450 system is a large and diverse group of enzymes that "metabolize" drugs as they enter the body; this system accounts for nearly 75 percent of the total number of metabolic reactions occurring within the body. As is noted by the pie chart below, there are "families" of CYP (usually called *substrates*) though which drugs are metabolized (Figure 5-1). If one drug is metabolized by one of the same families of CYP450, the net result may be either a net increase ("inhibitor") or decrease ("inducer") in the drug's concentration in the body; this process leads to a drug-drug interaction.

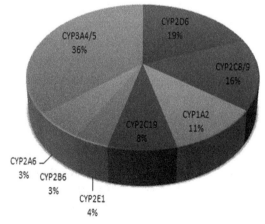

Figure 5-1. "Families" of the CYP450 system

This system is easily forgotten even by the most diligent practitioners, but it represents a major source of drug-drug interactions in the body.

Since this system affects the metabolic clearance of 75% of all manufactured drugs, it is important to understand it. As was discussed above, if one drug is metabolized by one of the same families of CYP450, the net result may be either an increase or decrease in this drug's concentration.

To understand this best, one must understand the concept of inhibitors and inducers. Inhibitors act to **block** the metabolic activity of one or more of the CYP450 enzymes. If the metabolic activity of a drug is blocked by another drug, the concentration of that drug will subsequently increase in the body. That is, if drug A inhibits drug B, then drug B's concentration level in the bloodstream will be higher because its metabolism is **blocked**.

For example, most practitioners understand that when patients use antibiotics with warfarin (Coumadin®), the international normalized ratio (INR) will increase and possibly become supratherapeutic. This process may occur as a result of the antibiotic "inhibiting" the metabolism of warfarin; that is, the body can't metabolize the warfarin as well, because the antibiotic **blocks** it's ability to get metabolized. This means an inhibitor can ultimately result in a clinically significant **increase** in pharmacologic effects of drugs.

On the other hand, some medications act as inducers, which **increase** the metabolic activity of one or more of the CYP450 enzymes. If a medication increases the metabolic activity of another medication, the drug is "cleared" from the body more rapidly. That is, if drug A induces drug B, then drug B's concentration level in the blood stream will be lower. This means an inducer can result in a clinically significant **decrease** in the pharmacological effect of the drug.

For example, the drug rifampin (drug A) acts as an inducer of warfarin (drug B). Consequently, if someone was using rifampin and warfarin together, the warfarin would be metabolized at an accelerated rate, and the patient would require more warfarin to get the same effect (i.e., a clinically significant **decrease** in warfarin levels). This patient is likely to require higher doses of warfarin to get the same therapeutic INR as a consequence of this concept of "inducers."

Table 5-1 is meant to illustrate the above: Drug A acts as either an inhibitor or an inducer of Drug B. The consequence is either a clinically significant increase in drug B or a clinically significant decrease in drug B (depending on whether it is an inhibitor or an inducer).

Table 5-1. Example of Inhibitors and Inducers

	Inhibitor	Inducer
Drug A	Bactrim DS®	rifampin
Drug B	Coumadin®	Coumadin®
Net Effect	Bactrim inhibits coumadin causing INR to increase	Rifampin inhibits coumadin causing INR to decrease

Table 5-2. Inhibitors - Cytochrome P450 (CYP) Enzymes Drug Table[21]

CYP1A2	CYP2B6	CYP2C8	CYP2C9	CYP2C19	CYP2D6	CYP2E1	CYP3A4
Amiodarone	Thiopeta	Anastrozole	Amiodarone	Cimetidine	Abiraterone	Disulfiram	Amiodarone
Atazanavir	Ticlopidine	Ezetmibe	Atazanavir	Citalopram	Amiodarone		Amprenavir
Cimetidine		Gemfibrozil	Cimetidine	Delavirdine	Asenapine		Aprepitant
Ciprofloxacin		Montelukast	Clopidogrel	Efavirenz	Buproprion		Atazanavir
Citalopram		Nicardipine	Cotrimloxazole	Felbamate	Celecoxib		Boceprevir Cimetidine
Clarithromycin		Sulfinpyrazone	Delavirdine	Fluconazole	Chloroquine		Ciprofloxacin
Diltiazem		Trimethoprim	Disulfram	Fluoxetine	Chlorpheniramine		Clarithromycin
Enoxacin			Efavirenz	Fluvastatin	Chlorpromazine		Cyclosporine
Erythromycin			Fenofibrate	Fluvoxamine	Cimetidine		Danazol
Estradiol			Fluconazole	Indomethacin	Cimacalcet		Delavirdine
Fluvoxamine			Fluorouracil	Isoniazid	Citalopram		Diltiazem
Interferon			Fluoxetine	Ketoconazole	Clemastine		Efavirenz
Isoniazid Ketoconazcle			Fluvastatin	Lansoprazole	Clomipramine		Erythromycin
Methoxsalen			Fluvoxamine	Modafinil	Cocaine		Ethinyl Estradiol
Mibefradil			Gemfibrozil	Omeprazole	Darifenacin		Ezetimibe (p)
Tegaserod			Imatinib	Oxcarbazepine	Desipramine		Fluconazole

32

Isoniazid
Itraconazole
Ketoconazole
Leftlunomide
Lovastatin
Methoxsalen
Metronidazole*
Mexiletine
Modafinil
Nalidixic acid
Norethindrone
Norfloxacin
Omeprazole
Contraceptives
Paroxetine
Phenylbutazone
Pfobenecid

Probenecid
Ticlodipine
Topiramate

Diphenhydramine
Doxepin
Doxorubicin
Duloxetine
Escitalopram
Febuxostat
Fluoxetine
Fluophenazine
Halofantrine
Haloperidol
Hydroxychloroquine
Hydroxyzine
Imatinib
Levomepromzine

Fluoxetine
Fluvoxamine
Gestodene
Imatinib
Indinavir
Isoniazid
Itraconazole
Ketoconazole*
Methylprednisolone
Mibefradil
Miconazole
Mifepristone
Nefazodone
Neltinavir
Nicardipine

Table 5-2 (continued). Inhibitors - Cytochrome P450 (CYP) Enzymes Drug Table[21]

CYP1A2	CYP2B6	CYP2C8	CYP2C9	CYP2C19	CYP2D6	CYP2E1	CYP3A4
See previous page	See previous page	See previous page	Continued from previous page	See previous page	Continued from previous page	See previous page	Continued from previous page
			Sertraline		Methadone		Norethindrone
					Metoclopramide		Norfloxacin
			Sulfaphenazole		Minefradil		Norfluoxetine
			Sulfonamides		Midodrine		Oxiconazole
			Tacrine		Moclobemide		Posaconazole
			Teniposide		Nefazodone		Prednisone
			Ticlodipine		Norfluoxetine		Quinine
			Tipranavir		Paroxetine		Ranolazine
			Troleandomycin		Perphenazine		Ritonavir
			Voriconazole		Propafenone		Saquinavir
			Zafirlukast		Propranolol		Sertraline
			Zileuton		Quinacrine		Telaprevir
					Quinidne		Telithromycin
					Ranitidine		Troleandomycin

Verapamil

Voriconazole

Zafirlukast

Zileutin

Ranolazine

Ritonavir

Sertraline

Tegaserod

Terbinafine

Thioridazine

Ticloodipine

Tipranavir

Tripelennamine

Reprinted with permission from Pharmacology Weekly.

Table 5-3. Inducers - Cytochrome P450 (CYP) Enzymes Drug Table[21]

CYP1A2	CYP2B6	CYP2C8	CYP2C9	CYP2C19	CYP2D6	CYP2E1	CYP3A4
Carbamazepine	Barbiturates	Carbamazepine	Aprepitant	Barbiturates	Carbamazepine	4-methylPyrazole	Amprenavir
Clotrimazole	Phenobarbital	Phenytoin	Barbiturates	Norethndrone	Ethanol	Ethanol	Barbiturates
Phenobarbital	Phenytoin	Rifabutin	Carbamazepine	Phenytoin	Phenobarbital	Isoniazid	Carbamazepine
Phenytoin	Primidone	Rifampin	Primidone	Rifampin	Phenytoin		Clotrimazole
Primidone	Roflumilast		Rifampin		Primidone		Dexamethasone
Psoralen			Vigabatrin		Rifampin		Efavirenz
Smoking							Ethosuximide
							Griseofulvin
							Modafinil
							Nevirapine
							Oxcarbazepine
							Phenobarbital
							Phenytoin
							Prednisone
							Primidone
							Rifambutin
							Rifampin
							Rifapentine
							Ritonavir
							Topiramate

Reprinted with permission from Pharmacology Weekly.

The lists in the preceding pages (Tables 5-2,3)[21] represents the more common *inhibitors* and *inducers* of prescribed medications. To say the least, the list is daunting. Part of the reason for this is the number of drugs that comes to market. In 2011, 30 new molecular entities (NMEs), or drugs that have never before been approved, were approved by the FDA.[22] Additionally, of the 30 new drugs that were brought to market, as well as those that already exist in the United States, there were 81 "new" FDA-approved uses for drugs.[23] On this basis, it is difficult (nearly impossible) to understand if a drug is either inhibited by or an inducer of other drugs. Simply looking at this list only complicates matters. However, since this is the site of drug-drug interactions, it is recommended that all providers have a firm understanding of common medications where interactions pose risk to patients.

The best way to evaluate for drug-drug interactions is through the newly integrated EHRs (Electronic Health Records), which include "drug-drug calculators" and are now mandated for the highest level of reimbursement in the healthcare system. Other techniques include discussion with pharmacists prior to prescribing. But perhaps the simplest technique is access to applications that nearly everyone can get on iPhone or Blackberry™ devices. These devices allow providers to plug in medications that a patient is taking and then cross-reference reactions that may occur when those drugs are taken in combination. It is perhaps one of the safest ways to minimize drug-drug interactions. Table 5-4 represents resources that providers and non-providers can use to check for drug-drug interactions.

Table 5-4. Resources to Check for Drug-Drug Interactions

http://www.epocrates.com
A FREE/or pay drug interaction checker that will display any interactions between your chosen drug(s). Available online and as an Application for smart-phone devices.
http://www.drugs.com/drug_interactions.html
A FREE drug interaction checker that will display any interactions between your chosen drug(s) and food. Available online only.
http://naturaldatabase.therapeuticresearch.com
A FREE herbal drug interaction checker that will display any interactions between your chosen herbal drugs. Available online only.
http://www.lexi.com
A purchasable drug interaction checker that will display any interactions between your chosen drug(s). Available online and as an application for smart-phone devices.

Table 5-5. Food Products and the CYP450 System

Type of products	Impact on CYP450
Avocado	inducer of CYP450
Broccoli	inducer of CYP450
Brussel sprouts	inducer of CYP450
Carrots, Celery	inducer of CYP450
Char-grilled meat	inducer of CYP450
Cranberry	inhibitor of CYP450
Grapefruit juice	potent inhibitor of CYP450
Soya	inhibitor of CYP450
St John's wort	inducer of CYP450

As can be seen in Table 5-5, CYP450-mediated activity can also be affected by certain dietary habits. As an example, grapefruit juice is known to inhibit CYP3A4-mediated metabolism and can inhibit certain medications like some statins. On the other hand, tobacco smoking has been known to induce CYP450 and thereby can have a significant impact on medications like olanzapine (Zyprexa®).

Let us discuss the latter of the two first. The clearance of olanzapine (Zyprexa®) is increased in smokers; that is, smoking acts as an inducer of olanzapine. In one study, smokers were found to increase the clearance of olanzapine by 98 percent.[24] The accelerated rate at which olanzapine is cleared by the CYP450 system means that, for a patient who smokes, the amount of olanzapine this patient takes would need to be increased in order to get the same effect.

However, what happens if the patient on olanzapine decides to quit? To elaborate with an example: a patient who smokes one pack per day comes into the hospital for acute change in condition; the facility is smoke free. His medication list shows that he takes olanzapine. During his stay he gets more confused for unknown reasons. Why?

Since the patient can no longer smoke, the inducer of the medication olanzapine is *no longer* present. Consequently, the levels of olanzapine will now rise in the blood stream since there is no inducer to accelerate its metabolism. This would explain why the patient had another acute change in his condition shortly after the admission. Advice for a patient who smokes and takes olanzapine might be to decrease the amount of olanzapine prior to the abstinence of smoking, then a subsequent decrease after he/she quits smoking. Another option would be to supplement the patient with a nicotine patch which induces the Zyprexa just as his/her cigarette smoking did.

Other circumstances of drug-drug interactions occur as a result of an enhanced (not inhibitory) effect of medications when taken together rather than interactions with CYP450. Examples of drugs with an enhanced drug effect are listed in Table 5-6 (not listed in order or importance).

ACE inhibitors have long been known for causing hyperkalemia. They may cause hyperkalemia because angiotensin II increases aldosterone release. Since aldosterone is responsible for increasing the excretion of potassium, ACE inhibitors ultimately cause retention of potassium.

The incidence of hyperkalemia can be as high as 9.8 percent when using ACE's.[25] This number should not deter providers from giving these medications, however, since they can be very effective for diseases like congestive heart failure (CHF) and diabetes mellitus (DM) to name a few. In the presence of potassium, ACE inhibitors can cause hyperkalemia. In the presence of spironolactone (Aldactone®), ACE inhibitors can also result in abnormal serum potassium levels. The combination, albeit very important and even *necessary* in many disease states, can lead to an enhanced effect of hyperkalemia. As stated earlier, 95 percent of all ADEs are predictable. The enhanced effects of ACE's and spironolactone or potassium are also predictable. Monitoring frequently (in 3-6 month increments) would likely be sufficient to safely treat older adults, but knowing that the risk exists is, by far, the best predictor for minimizing an adverse drug event.

ACE inhibitors in combination with non-steroidal anti-inflammatory drugs (NSAIDs), or ACE inhibitors in the presence of spironolactone as discussed earlier, can lead to renal insufficiency, or worse, acute renal failure (ARF). Again, the risk is present and important, but a practitioner who knows this risk exists also decreases the risk of an adverse event from occurring.

Aspirin (ASA) with NSAIDs increases the risk of peptic ulcers. Older adults have a greater likelihood of GI hemorrhage than do younger adults due to physiological factors. Using these two medications together, however, markedly increases the risk of GI bleeding.

A commonly overlooked enhanced effect occurs with patients who take benzodiazepines. Any "benzo" (PRN or routinely) in the presence of certain antidepressants and antipsychotics can result in increased sedation and delirium or confusion. The biggest risk for the use of these medications together is falls. In the elderly, any medication that increases the risk of falls should be avoided unless otherwise necessary.

Carbamazepine (Tegretol®) can be inhibited by several drugs. In the presence of inhibitors, as was discussed earlier, Tegretol levels may increase in the blood stream. Therefore, any patient on routine prescriptions of those inhibitors (*as noted at the bottom of Table 5-6*) should have frequent follow-up checks of Tegretol levels.

Table 5-6. Drugs Interactions with Enhanced Drug Effects

Drug A	Drug B	Effect(s)
ACE inhibitors	NSAIDs, spironolactone, potassium	Hyperkalemia / Renal insufficiency / ARF
ASA (aspirin)	NSAIDs	Peptic ulcers
Benzodiazepine	antidepressant	Sedation; confusion; falls
Benzodiazepine	antipsychotic	Sedation; confusion; falls
Carbamazepine	Enzyme Inhibitors*	Increased levels of drug A
Corticosteroids	NSAIDs/ASA	Peptic ulcers
Digoxin	Amiodorone, diltiazem, verapamil	Increased digoxin effects (arrhythmia)
Digoxin	Diuretics	Arrhythmia, dehydration, electrolyte imbalance
Lithium	NSAIDs, thiazide diuretics	Increased lithium levels
Phenothiazines	Antihistamines and TCAs	Increase anti-cholinergic effects
Phenytoin	Enzyme inhibitors*	Increased phenytoin levels
Quinolones	NSAIDs	Seizure threshold is decreased
Theophylline	Enzyme Inhibitors* / Quinolones	Increased theophylline levels

*Enzyme inhibitors: amiodorone, fluconazole, ketoconazole, erythromycin, clarithromycin, sulfa's, cimetidine, ciprofloxacin

Corticosteroids have several side effects, but one of the more important is that it weakens the lining of the stomach. Consequently, there is an increased risk of GI bleed in patients using corticosteroids. Use of corticosteroids with NSAIDs and ASA substantially increases the risk of peptic ulcers and GI bleeding associated with it.

Digoxin taken with either amiodorone, diltiazem, or verapamil has been known to increase digoxin effects. Should these medications be used in combination, it is imperative that digoxin levels be followed quarterly to semi-annually (or sooner if the provider deems it important). In general, digoxin has long been known to be risky in older adults. Chapters 6 and 7 will elaborate on this risk.

Additionally, digoxin in the presence of diuretics (especially loop diuretics) can lead to either electrolyte imbalances, arrhythmias, or dehydration. It is recommended that any older adult using diuretics in the presence of digoxin be frequently monitored for dehydration and electrolyte imbalances, since they can lead to serious and occasionally lethal arrhythmias.

Lithium, which has a very narrow therapeutic range, should be avoided in the presence of diuretics (e.g., lasix, hydrochlorothiazide, chlorthalidone) as they are known to increase serum lithium levels. NSAIDs too can have the same effect on serum lithium levels, so they should be avoided by those patients who take lithium.

Phenothiazines (Thorazine, Compazine, Phenergan), when mixed with antihistamines, over-the-counter and prescribed, or tricyclic antidepressants enhance the anticholinergic side effects of the "thiazine." Anticholinergic agents are best known for their effects on worsening cognition, but the mnemonic "no see, no spit, no pee, no sh!&" is another way of remembering the deleterious effects of anticholinergic agents.

Of all the medications prescribed to patients in the U.S. market, the most common and most likely to remain on patients' med-lists for the continuum of their lives are seizure medications. Phenytoin (Dilantin®) has been used for a very long time to help control seizure disorders, but Dilantin has a very narrow therapeutic range that must be checked frequently. In geriatric adults there is also a concern that Dilantin will interact with other medications and lead to a drug-drug interaction. Dilantin is inhibited by amiodorone, fluconazole, ketoconazole, erythromycin, clarithromycin, sulfa drugs, cimetidine, and a very common antibiotic used in geriatric adult medicine, ciprofloxacin. Today there are better and safer alternatives than Dilantin; lamotrigine (Lamictal®) and levetiracetam (Keppra®) are examples and should be encouraged to minimize drug-drug interactions.

Just as there are medications that can have enhanced drug effects when used in combination with other medications, there also are drugs that can have a reduced effect when used in combination with other medications (Table 5-7). This warning should not be confused with inducers as described earlier.

Table 5-7. Drug Interactions with Reduced Drug Effects

Drug A	Drug B	Effect(s)
Anti-HTN agents (ACE, thiazides, beta-blockers)	NSAIDs	Reduced effects of Drug A
Digoxin	Cholestyramine	Reduced effects of Drug A
Quinolones	Cholestyramine	Reduced effects of Drug A

All NSAIDs (including cox-2's like Celebrex®) increase the likelihood of elevating a patient's blood pressure. NSAIDs in any form are not recommended in geriatric adults, but if they are used, practitioners should EXPECT an elevation of blood pressure. This is true even in the presence of blood pressure medications. Therefore, all anti-hypertensive agents (ACE's, thiazides, beta-blockers) will have a reduced drug effect in the presence of NSAIDs.

Cholestyramine (Questran®) was originally prescribed to reduce cholesterol levels but is rarely used for this since the advent of statins. Today, you may see this medication used for one of the side effects it causes: constipation. This drug would be effective if someone was having diarrhea; however, if a medication is given with Questran, practitioners should expect a decrease in the absorption and efficacy of that medication. As a general rule with Questran, avoid administering other medications within one hour of, or 4 hours after, a dose is given. Two of the common examples (*in Table 5-7*) are digoxin and the class of antibiotics known as *quinolones* (Levaquin®, ciprofloxacin, Floxin®, and Avelox®). The effects of either one of these medications, if given with Questran, will be reduced.

Warfarin is another medication that has many drug-drug interactions. Even though warfarin is inhibited or induced by nearly all medications, pharmacodynamic antagonism or synergism may also affect INR levels. Table 5-8 details the effects of other medications in the presence of warfarin.

Table 5-8. Drug Interactions with Warfarin

Interacting Drug	Effect	INR Effects
Cholestyramine	Reduced anticoagulant effect	INR decreases
Barbiturates, carbamazepine, phenytoin*, primidone, rifampin	Reduced anticoagulant effect	INR decreases
Amiodorone, cimetidine, ciprofloxacin, clarithromycin, e-mycin, fluconazole, itraconazole, ketoconazole, metronidazole, sulfonamides, thyroxine, gemfibrozil, phenytoin**, salicylates, tamoxifen	Increased anti-coagulation effect	INR increases
NSAIDs	Increased risk of bleeding	INR usually increases
Oral contraceptives (not in Geriatrics), vitamin K	anticoagulant effect	INR usually decreases

*phenytoin effects reduces anti-coagulation effect by inducing warfarin metabolism

** phenytoin enhances warfarin's effects by pharmacodynamic potentiation of anticoagulation effect

Most drugs increase the anticoagulation effect of warfarin and thereby increase the INR, but some medications (mostly anti-seizure medications) will reduce the anticoagulation effect. Carbamazepine (Tegretol®), pheytoin (Dilantin®), Primidone (Mysoline®) and many barbiturates (phenobarbitol) will reduce the anticoagulation effect, making it more difficult to get INRs to therapeutic ranges.

Top Ten Dangerous Drug Interactions

In fact, because warfarin interacts with so many medications, it should not surprise providers that it is listed on the top ten dangerous drug interactions list. The list below describes which medications have the most significant drug-drug interactions followed by a description of the interaction. Fifty percent of the time, warfarin makes the list.

- Warfarin — NSAIDs
- Warfarin — Sulfa drugs
- Warfarin — Macrolides
- Warfarin — Quinolones
- Warfarin — Phenytoin
- ACE inhibitors — Potassium supplements
- ACE inhibitors — Spironolactone
- Digoxin — Amiodarone
- Digoxin — Verapamil
- Theophylline — Quinolones (ciprofloxacin, norfloxacin, oflaxacin)

Examples:

Warfarin > NSAIDs (doesn't include Celebrex)
- *may increase INR*
- *increases risk of GI bleeding*

Warfarin > Sulfonamides (Bactrim®, Septra®, sulfamethoxazole)
- *increases INR, increasing risk of bleeding*

Warfarin > Macrolides (Biaxin®, erythromycin, Zithromax®)
- *increases INR, increasing risk of bleeding*

Warfarin > Quinolones (Avelox®, Cipro®, Floxin®, Levaquin®, Noroxin®)
- *increases INR, increasing risk of bleeding*

Warfarin > Phenytoin (Dilantin®)
- *may increase or decrease INR*

ACE inhibitors (Accupril®, Altace®, Capoten®, lisinopril, Lotensin®, Univasc®) > **Potassium**
- *increases risk of hyperkalemia*

ACE inhibitors (Accupril®, Altace®, Capoten®, lisinopril, Lotensin®, Univasc®) > **Aldactone**
- *increases risk of hyperkalemia*

digoxin > amiodorone
- *combination may increase digoxin levels leading to toxicity and cardiac side effects*

digoxin > verapamil
- *combination may increase digoxin levels leading to toxicity*
- *increases risk of AV block*

theophylline > Quinolones (only Cipro®, Floxin®, Noroxin®)
- *combination may increase theophylline levels*

What about drug-drug interactions among over-the-counter (OTC) drugs? Table 5-9 describes common reactions that occur with OTC agents. The risks of over-the-counter medications have long been known but commonly occur because older adults are either not informed about the risks of OTC medications, or assume there is little risk because they are OTC medications.

Acetaminophen (Tylenol®), when used with rifampin, can potentiate the effects of Tylenol® as it is metabolized through the liver, potentiating acetaminophen toxicity and liver failure. If the combination is given, practitioners should limit the dosing of Tylenol® to less than the current recommendation of 3000 milligrams. Recommendation: No more than 2 grams.

Table 5-9. Drug-Drug Interactions of Common OTC Drugs

OTC Drug	Prescription Drug or Class	Adverse Effect
Acetaminophen (APAP)	Rifampin	Potentiates APAP effects resulting in liver failure
NSAIDs	Methotrexate	Can increase methotrexate levels
NSAIDs	Digoxin, beta-blockers, diuretics	Reduces BP lowering effects
NSAIDs	Warfarin	NSAIDs increase blood-thinning effect of blood thinners
Ibuprofen; Naproxen sodium	Lithium	Lithium toxicity
Antihistamines (brompheniramine, chlorpheniramine, dimenhydrinate, diphenhydramine, doxylamine)	Alprazolam, temazepam	Increased sedation/lethargy
Pseudoephedrine	MAOI's (phenelzine, selegiline, tranylcypromine)	Life-threatening arrhythmia's
Dextromethorphan	SSRIs ; MAOIs	Serotonin syndrome
Dextromethorphan	Sedatives	Increased sedation/lethargy

Any NSAID, when used with methotrexate can increase the serum methotrexate levels. In addition, any patient using anti-hypertensives should clearly understand that all NSAIDs decrease the blood-pressure lowering effects for any blood pressure medication. Furthermore, NSAIDs when used with warfarin (Coumadin®) can result in supratherapeutic INRs and thereby increase the risks of hemorrhage. Finally, NSAIDs in combination with lithium can potentiate the effects of lithium leading to toxicity; NSAIDs should be avoided in patients using lithium.

A common interaction occurs when patients use benzodiazepines, such as alprazolam or temazepam, with OTC cold remedies. Common antihistamines that can be found in nearly all OTC "cold" products include: brompheniramine, chlorpheniramine, dimenhydrinate, diphenyhydramine, doxylamine. In combination, older adults can become seriously, even lethally, over-sedated.

Another dangerous and potentially life-threatening interaction is pseudoephedrine with monoamine oxidase inhibitors (MAOIs). MAOIs are a class of antidepressants usually prescribed by psychiatrists. Besides psychiatrists, neurologists might also prescribe these medications, particularly for patients with Parkinson's disease. A common MAOI inhibitor used by neurologists is selegiline. Any practitioner who comes across a patient taking an MAOI must pay careful attention to other medications being used with it in order to avoid serious drug-drug interactions that usually result in life-threatening arrhythmias.

Dextromethorphan can also interact dangerously with MAOIs. Any patient taking MAOIs must be informed that dextromethorphan is very dangerous, and potentially lethal, with these products. Additionally, dextromethorphan is likely to increase sedation when used with any sedative or narcotic agent. Finally, when MAOIs are taken with SSRIs (Lexapro®, Celexa®, Zoloft®), the result can lead to a *serotonin syndrome.*

Serotonin syndrome is a potentially life threatening drug reaction that causes the body to have too much serotonin. Symptoms can occur within minutes and as late as several hours later. Symptoms include:

- Agitation or restlessness
- Nausea, Vomiting, Diarrhea
- Tachycardia
- Hallucinations
- Hyperthermia
- Loss of coordination
- Overactive reflexes
- Rapid changes and fluctuations in blood pressure
- Seizures

Chapter 6
The "Beers List"

As stated earlier, the Beers Criteria was developed as a tool to identify inappropriate drugs or high-risk drugs in the elderly. The tables that follow will list inappropriate drugs in the elderly as originally detailed by Beers and colleagues.[21] The newest update to the Beers Criteria occurred in 2012, and this is the fourth revision to the list since it was released. This latest update includes new evidence of potentially inappropriate medications for the elderly, grading of each recommendation by the strength and quality of studies to suggest why it should make the list, and, finally, exceptions to the criteria.

Although the Beers Criteria is an invaluable tool when prescribing for older patients, one major difference between this and previous publications is that the Criteria should not substitute for professional judgment or dictate prescribing for any patient when the practitioner believes that benefits of the medication(s) outweigh the potential risks. Simply put, the "Beers List" is not applicable in every circumstance. For example, a clinician prescribing for an individual receiving end-of-life or palliative care might determine a medication that may be potentially inappropriate for older adults, but realistically, is the only and most reasonable choice for that individual.

The 11-panelists note, "If a provider is not able to find an alternative and chooses to continue to use a drug on the list in an individual patient, designation of the medication as potentially inappropriate can serve as a reminder for close monitoring so that [adverse drug effects] can be incorporated into the electronic health record and prevented or detected early."[26] The Criteria are not meant to be used punitively, but rather, to inform clinical decision making, research, and training to improve the quality and safety of prescribing for older adults.

The table below (Table 6-1) describes the quality and strength of the evidence used in the updated version of the Beer Criteria.[26.]

Table 6-1. Designations of Quality and Strength of Evidence

Designation	Description
Quality of Evidence	
High	Evidence includes consistent results from well-designed, well-conducted studies in representative populations that directly assess effects on health outcomes (≥2 consistent, higher-quality randomized controlled trials or multiple consistent observational studies without no significant methodological flaws showing large effects).
Moderate	Evidence is sufficient to determine effects on health outcomes, but the number, quality, size or consistency of include studies; generalizability to routine practice; or indirect nature of the evidence of health outcomes (≥1 higher-quality trial with >100 participants; ≥ 2 higher quality trials with some inconsistency; ≥2 consistent, lower-quality trials; or multiple, consistent observational studies with no significant methodological flaws showing at least moderate effects) limits the strength of evidence.
Low	Evidence is sufficient to assess effects on health outcomes because of limited number or power of studies, large and unexplained inconsistency between higher-quality studies, important flaws in study design or conduct, gaps in the chain of evidence, or lack of information on important health outcomes.
Strength of Recommendation	
Strong	Benefits outweigh risks and burden OR risk and burden clearly outweigh benefits.
Weak	Benefits finely balanced with risks and burden.
Insufficient	Insufficient evidence to determine net benefits or risks.

(AGS Updated Beers Criteria for Potentially Inappropriate Medication Use in Older Adults (2012), www.americangeriatrics.org)

Previous versions of the Beers list have included appropriate criticisms about the quality of evidence used to discuss why certain medications "made the list" while others were "left off." In addition, the list seemingly served to penalize practitioners without knowledge behind the appropriateness of the medication in question.

As stated before, this panel consisted of 11 experts in geriatric care and pharmacology who both "graded" and performed a systematic review of each medication selected. At least one member on the board explains that the panel meant the list to be a guide to avoid inappropriate prescribing and *NOT* as a tool to penalize any practitioner. Consequently, the list included not only *potentially* inappropriate medications but also classes of medications to avoid in older adults. It also included medications to avoid in older adults with certain syndromes and/or diseases that might exacerbate certain conditions. Finally, it included medications that are "cautionary" for older adults.

The following Tables (6-2; 6-4–6-12) detail ALL of the medications included in Beers Criteria. However, the discussions that follow each table will include only medications that practitioners may commonly see. A free reference/pocket card format of the Beers Criteria can be retrieved at:

http://www.americangeriatrics.org/files/documents/beers/
PrintableBeersPocketCard.pdf

Table 6-2. Anticholinergics (First Generation Antihistamines)

Organ System or Therapeutic Category or Drug	Rationale	Recommendation	Quality/ Strength
First-generation antihistamines brompheniramine carbinoxamine* chlorpheniramine clemastine cyproheptadine dexbrompheniramine* dexchlorpheniramine* diphenhydramine (oral) doxylamine hydroxyzine promethazine triprolidine*	Highly anticholinergic; clearance reduced with advanced age, and tolerance develops when used as hypnotic; greater risk of confusion, dry mouth, constipation, and other anticholinergic effects and toxicity. Use of diphenhydramine in special situations such as acute treatment of severe allergic reaction may be appropriate.	Avoid	Hydroxyzine and promethazine high; all others moderate/ strong

*New on 2012 American Geriatrics Society Updated Beers Criteria

(AGS Updated Beers Criteria for Potentially Inappropriate Medication Use in Older Adults (2012), www.americangeriatrics.org)

First generation antihistamines are commonly found as over-the-counter agents nowadays. Common examples include diphyenyhydramine (Bendaryl®), chlorpheniramine (Chlor-Trimeton®) and doxylamine (Unisom®). Other first generation antihistamines are prescribed: cyproheptadine (Periactin®), hydroxyzine (Atarax®), promethazine (Phenergan®).

All first-generation antihistamines are highly anticholinergic with side effects that can be remembered with the phrase "no see, no spit, no pee, no sh!&." More appropriately, however, anticholinergic agents are infamous for causing "anti-SLUD." This acronym includes the main features of anticholinergic agents: anti-salivation, anti-lacrimation, anti-urination and anti-defecation. Table 6-3 shows all of the dangerous and serious side effects of anticholinergic agents.

Table 6-3. Symptoms of Anticholinergic Drugs

Physical Symptoms	Cognitive Symptoms
Blurred vision Hot, dry skin / dehydration Dry mouth Shortness of breath Dilated pupils Increased heart rate Increased / decreased psychomotor activity Anorexia Urinary Retention	Confusion / clouding of consciousness Memory impairment Visual hallucinations Sensory illusions Disturbance in sleep-wake cycle Disorientation, especially to time and place Incoherent speech Anxiety, agitation, excitement

As can clearly be seen, both the physical and cognitive side effects of these agents are quite severe and explain, quite simply, why these agents should be avoided when feasible.

Any anticholinergic drug has reduced clearance in those with advanced age. And, when these medications are used as sleep aids, tolerance develops requiring higher and higher doses to achieve the same effect, which eventually risks toxicity. On the other hand, Bendaryl can, and perhaps even should, be used in situations such as acute treatment of severe allergic reactions.

The recommendation, as described in the Beers Criteria, is to generally avoid first-generation antihistamines in geriatric adults. The quality of evidence to support this is "high" for hydroxyzine and promethazine, and the quality of evidence for all the others in its class is considered moderate.

Other anticholinergic agents are antiparkinson's agents (Table 6-4). Two of the agents that made the Beers Criteria include benztropine (Cogentin®) and trihexyphenidyl (Artane®). Both are used for parkinsonisms or extrapyramidal reactions that may occur with drugs used to control features associated with Parkinson's disease or parkinsonisms. Nowadays, more effective agents than the ones described here are available; therefore, the recommendation in geriatrics is to avoid them. The quality of evidence is moderate, and the strength of that recommendation is strong.

Table 6-4. Anticholinergics (Antiparkinson Agents)

Organ System or Therapeutic Category or Drug	Rationale	Recommendation	Quality/ Strength
Benztropine	Not recommended for prevention of EPS with antipsychotics,; mor-effective agents available for treatment of Parkinson's.	**AVOID**	Moderate / Strong
Trihexyphenidyl*			

*New on 2012 American Geriatrics Society Updated Beers Criteria

(AGS Updated Beers Criteria for Potentially Inappropriate Medication Use in Older Adults (2012), www.americangeriatrics.org).

Additional anticholinergic agents include drugs used for GI tract spasms: a class of medications called antispasmodics (Table 6-5). Common examples include belladona alkaloids (Donnatal®), dicyclomine (Bentyl®), hyoscyamine (Levsin®), and scopolamine (Scopace®). These medications tend to be very anticholinergic but have uncertain effectiveness. The general recommendation in geriatrics is to avoid them; however, there may be some clinical benefits short-term for those patients in palliative or hospice care. The quality of evidence that exists for the antispasmodics is moderate while the strength of the recommendation is strong.

Table 6-5. Anticholinergics (Antispasmodics)

Organ System or Therapeutic Category or Drug	Rationale	Recommendation	Quality/ Strength
Belladonna alkaloids Trihexyphenidyl* Clidinium-chlordiazepoxide* Dicyclomine Hyoscyamine Propantheline* Scopolamine	Highly anti-cholinergic, uncertain effectiveness.	Avoid **EXCEPT** in short-term palliative care to decrease oral secretions	Moderate / Strong

*New on 2012 American Geriatrics Society Updated Beers Criteria

(AGS Updated Beers Criteria for Potentially Inappropriate Medication Use in Older Adults (2012), www.americangeriatrics.org).

Two antithrombotics have been placed on Beers 2012 (Table 6-6). Dipyridamole (Persantine®) in the oral short-acting form was placed on the list because it has been known to cause orthostatic hypotension. It is important to note that both the IV form and the long-acting formulation are still acceptable for use in patients undergoing a cardiac stress test. Ticlopidine (Ticlid®) is the second agent. The quality of evidence to support the recommendation is moderate while the strength behind the recommendation is strong.

Table 6-6. Anticholinergics (Antithrombotics)

Organ System or Therapeutic Category or Drug	Rationale	Recommendation	Quality/ Strength
Dipyridamole* (oral short-acting)	May cause orthostatic hypotension; more-effective alternatives available; IV form acceptable for use in cardiac stress test.	Avoid	Moderate / Strong
Ticlopidine	Safer effective alternatives available.	Avoid	Moderate / Strong

*New on 2012 American Geriatrics Society Updated Beers Criteria

(AGS Updated Beers Criteria for Potentially Inappropriate Medication Use in Older Adults (2012), www.americangeriatrics.org).

The anti-infective agent nitrofurantoin (Macrodantin®/Macrobid®) is the only anti-effective agent on Beers 2012 (Table 6-7). It has long been known that Macrodbid® increases the potential for pulmonary toxicity (diffuse interstitial pneumonitis or pulmonary fibrosis, or both), and it increases after the agent is used for a chronic period of time. It is best to avoid for long-term suppression. In addition, it is best to avoid with patients with a GFR < 60mL/min/1.73m^2 since a strong concentration in the urine is required for the drug to work effectively.

Table 6-7. Anti-infectives

Organ System or Therapeutic Category or Drug	Rationale	Recommendation	Quality/ Strength
Nitrofurantoin*	Potential for pulmonary toxicity; safer alternatives available; lack of efficacy in patients with low GFR due to inadequate drug concentration in the urine.	Avoid for long-term suppression; avoid in patients with low GFR	Moderate / Strong

*New on 2012 American Geriatrics Society Updated Beers Criteria

Adapted from (AGS Updated Beers Criteria for Potentially Inappropriate Medication Use in Older Adults (2012), www.americangeriatrics.org).

Since cardiovascular agents (Table 6-8) make up the bulk of drugs that have the highest frequency of ADE's (*see Chapter 4*), it shouldn't be surprising that these agents make up the bulk of medications on the Beers Criteria.

Table 6-8 Cardiovascular Agents

Organ System or Therapeutic Category or Drug	Rationale	Recommendation	Quality/ Strength
Alpha, blockers: doxazosin prazosin* terazosin*	High risk of orthostatic Avoid use as an antihypertensive hypotension; not recommended as routine treatment for HTN; alternative agents have superior risk/benefit profile.	**Avoid** use as an antihypertensive	Moderate/ Strong
Alpha agonists, central clonidine guanabenz* guanfacine* methyldopa reserpine (>.lmg/ d)*	High risk of adverse CNS effects; may cause bradycardia and orthostatic hypotension; not recommended as routine treatment for hypertension.	**Avoid** clonidine as a first-line antihypertensive. Avoid others as listed.	Low/ Strong *(Continued)*

56

Table 6-8 (continued). Cardiovascular Agents

Organ System or Therapeutic Category or Drug	Rationale	Recommendation	Quality/Strength
Antiorrhythic drugs amiodarone dofetilide* dronedarone* flecainide* ibutilide* procainamide propafenone quinidine sotalol*	Data suggest that rate control yields better balance of benefits and harms (than rhythm control) for most older adults. Amiodorone is associated with multiple toxicities, including thyroid disease, pulmonary disorders, and QT-interval prolongation.	**Avoid** antiarrhythmic drugs as first-line treatment of atrial fibrillation.	Moderate/ Strong
Disopyramide	Potent negative inotrope and may induce heart failure in older adults; strongly anticholinergic; other antiarrythmic drugs preferred.	**Avoid**	Low/ Strong
Dronedarone*	High risk of orthostatic hypotension; not recommended as routine tx for hypertension; alternative agents have superior risk/ benefit profile.	**Avoid** in patients with permanent atrial fibrillation	Moderate/ Strong
Digoxin >0.12Smg/ day	In heart failure, higher dosages associated with no additional benefit and may increase risk of toxicity; slow renal clearance may led to risk of toxic effects.	**Avoid**	Low/ Strong
Nifedipine, immediate release	Potential for hypotension; risk of precipitating myocarial ischemia.	**Avoid**	High/ Strong
Sipronolactone (>25mg/day)	In heart failure, the risk of hyperkalemia is higher in older adults, especialy if taking > 25mg/day or taking condomitant NSAID, ACE, ARB or K+	**Avoid** in patients with heart failure or with low GFR	Moderate/ Strong

*New on 2012 American Geriatrics Society Updated Beers Criteria

(AGS Updated Beers Criteria for Potentially Inappropriate Medication Use in Older Adults (2012), www.americangeriatrics.org)

All of the alpha$_1$ blockers risk orthostatic hypotension and must be used in caution with any older adult. Not only do they relax certain muscles (such as in the prostate), but they keep the small peripheral blood vessels open. Blocking the effect of the blood vessels' ability to constrict, in effect, causes the vessels to permanently remain open and relaxed, even when a person needs an increase in blood pressures, such as when standing up. Since alternative anti-hypertensive agents have superior risk/benefit profiles, the benefit should outweigh the risk if the practitioner decides to use these agents. Incidentally, make note that in Beers 2012, they are referencing alpha$_1$ blockers as they relate to blood pressure management and not for enlargement of the prostate. Needless to say, if they are used for hyperplasia of the prostate, the practitioner should always consider how it might affect the patient's blood pressure. The quality of evidence to support this recommendation is moderate, and the strength of the recommendation is strong.

In addition, many of the central acting alpha-agonists, clonidine (Catapress®) probably being one of the most common (Table 6-8), also risk severe orthostatic hypotension; as such, these types of anti-hypertensives are implicated in many falls. Additionally, in geriatric adults, they have been implicated in adverse CNS effects, such as delirium, and in cardiac effects such as bradycardia. The strength of the recommendation is strong, and the quality of evidence has been shown to be low.

Antiarrhythmic agents pose a significant risk to patients who already have a high incidence of cardiac issues. The overuse of amiodarone in the geriatric population is one of the most common examples. Although it is true that amiodarone has been shown to be an effective antiarrhythmic medication for the maintenance of sinus rhythm, its use is limited by significant non-cardiovascular toxicities such as thyroid disease, pulmonary disorders, and QT-interval prolongation. In addition, the half-life ranges between 40-60 days, which poses additional risk to older adults. Randomized trials comparing "rate control" vs. "rhythm control" strategies for the treatment of atrial fibrillation have demonstrated that maintenance of sinus rhythm yields little to no added improvement in mortality.[27] More importantly, quality of life achieved little to no benefit over the rate control approach.[28] The medications in this list should be avoided unless the benefit outweighs the risk. The quality of evidence and the strength of this recommendation are strong.

Digoxin in doses greater than 125mcg has been associated with no additional benefit in patients with heart failure.[29] Digoxin also risks toxicity, especially considering the risk of toxic effects and slow renal clearance in adults who already experience impaired renal clearance. For patients who are on doses higher than 125mcg, it is recommended to support the benefit of this therapy over the risk; one way to do this is to ask cardiology to support the recommendation.

Nifedipine (immediate release) has long been known to increase the risk of hypotension; it has also been known to precipitate myocardial ischemia.[30] Both of those risks are now part of the package insert for nifedipine (Adalat® and Procardia®), and it is recommended to avoid this agent for treatment of immediate hypertension. It is important to note, however, that this recommendation does not apply to the long-acting formulation.

Spironolactone (Aldactone®) in doses greater than 25mg/day has also been placed on the 2012 Beers Criteria. Although Aldactone has some very distinct benefits in congestive heart failure, the risk of hyperkalemia is especially high as this agent is potassium-sparing.[31] This risk increases if patients are taking concomitant NSAIDs, ACE inhibitors, ARBs, or potassium.

Table 6-9. Agents Affecting the Central Nervous System

Organ System or Therapeutic Category or Drug	Rationale	Recommendation	Quality/ Strength
Tertiary TCAs			
amitriptyline chlordiazepoxide- amitriptyline clomipramine doxepin > 6mg/day imipramine perphenazine- amitriptyline trimipramine*	High risk of orthostatic hypotension. Avoid use as an antihypertensive; not recommended as routine treatment for HTN; alternative agents have superior risk/ benefit profile.	**Avoid**	High/ Strong
Antipsychotics, first (conventional) and second (atypical) generation	Increase risk of CVA and mortality in persons with dementia.	**Avoid**	Moderate/ Strong
Thioridazine Mesoridazine	Highly anticholinergic and risk of QT-interval prolongation.	**Avoid**	Moderate/ Strong
Barbituates			
amobarbital* butabarbital* butalbital* mephobarbital* pentobarbital* phenobarbital secobarbital*	High rate of physical dependence; tolerance to sleep benefits; risk of overdose at low dosages.	**Avoid**	High/ Strong

(Continued)

Table 6-9 (continued). Cardiovascular Agents

Organ System or Therapeutic Category or Drug	Rationale	Recommendation	Quality/ Strength
Benzodiazepines (short/intermediate acting) alprazolam estazolam ' lorazepam oxazepam ' temazepam triazolam *Benzodiazepines (long acting)* clorazepate* chlordiazepoxide-amitriptyline clidinium-chlordiazepoxide clonazepam diazepam flurazepam quazepam	Older adults have increased sensitivity to BZDs and slower metabolism of long-acting agents. In general, all BZDs increase risk of cognitive impairment, delirium, falls, fractures, and motor vehicle accidents In older adults. May be appropriate for seizure disorders, rapid eye movement sleep disorders, benzo withdrawal, ethanol withdrawal, severe generalized anxiety disorder, periprocedural anesthesia, end-of-life.	**Avoid** BZDs (any type) for treatment of insomnia, agitation, or delirium	High/ Strong
Chloral hydrate"	Tolerance occurs within 10 days and risks outweigh benefits in light of overdose with doses only 3 times the recommended doses.	**Avoid**	Low/ Strong
Meprobamate	High rate of physical dependence; very sedating.	**Avoid**	Moderate/ Strong

(Continued)

Table 6-9 (continued). Agents Affecting the Central Nervous System

Organ System or Therapeutic Category or Drug	Rationale	Recommendation	Quality/ Strength
Nonbenzodiazepine hypnotics	BZD-receptor agoinists that have adverse events similar to those of BZDs in older adults (delirium, falls, fractures); minimal improvement in sleep latency and duration.	Avoid chronic use (>90 days)	High/ Strong
eszopiclone* zolpidem* zaleplon*"			
Ergot mesylates* Isoxsuprine*	Lack of efficacy.	Avoid	High/ Strong

*New on 2012 American Geriatrics Society Updated Beers Criteria

(AGS Updated Beers Criteria for Potentially Inappropriate Medication Use in Older Adults (2012), www.americangeriatrics.org))

Delirium in the presence of medications that affect the central nervous system is quite common. Clinical experience has clearly shown that delirium in older adults can initiate, or otherwise be a key component in, a cascade of events that lead to a downward spiral of permanent functional decline, loss of independence, institutionalization, and death. Delirium affects an estimated 14–56% of all hospitalized elderly patients.[32] The Beers Criteria clearly acknowledge the implications of agents that affect mental state. The medications listed in Table 6-9 should be considered carefully to determine if they are indeed appropriate for geriatric adults.

Tertiary tricyclic antidepressants (TCAs) have long been used for sleep disorders and depression. The rationale for their placement on the Beers Criteria is they are highly anticholinergic (see Table 6-3). Also, all TCAs are known to cause orthostatic hypotension posing significant risks to older adults.[33] There are much safer and, frankly, better alternatives to these agents. In general, avoid these agents, but should patients be on them, strong considerations should be made to both reduce (abrupt discontinuance should be avoided) and discontinue these agents. The quality of evidence for this recommendation is high and has been demonstrated repeatedly. The strength of the evidence to support it is strong. Both first- and second-generation antipsychotic agents have long been known to pose significant risks to older adults. They do provide off-label benefit in the presence of dementia with behaviors in some circumstances, but all are known to increase the risk of stroke and mortality in patients who are older and demented.[33] Additionally, they risk hyperglycemia and diabetes, hyperlipidemia, and falls.

Thioridazine, better known as Mellaril®, is a typical antipsychotic belonging to the phenothiazine drug class. It is highly anticholinergic and has been associated with QT-prolongation. In addition, Mellaril has been associated with serious extrapyramidal symptoms.

It should be quite clear why barbiturates are listed on the Beers Criteria. All barbiturates, but particularly those listed, have a high rate of physical dependence and tolerance. More importantly, there is a risk of overdose, even at low dosages. They should be avoided in geriatrics adults.

All of the short-, intermediate-, and long-acting benzodiazepines risk cognitive impairment, delirium, and falls in the older patient. The most important risk is fractures that can occur when these medications are prescribed.[34] There is no doubt that these medications play a very important *beneficial* role when patients are at risk of harming themselves or others, and they require control of that behavior. However, these medications should be used prudently and, most importantly, in as short of a course as possible! It should be noted, though, that these medications are appropriate and necessary in the setting of seizure disorders, benzodiazepine withdrawal, ethanol withdrawal, periprocedural anesthesia, and care at the end-of-life. They can also be used routinely for *severe* generalized anxiety disorder (GAD) should other psychological treatments (pharmacological and non-pharmacological) fail. As an example, other safer agents (such as SSRIs and SNRIs) should be considered since long-term management with benzodiazepines can lead, over time, to tolerance and dependence.

Chloral hydrate is produced from chlorine and ethanol; in essence it is a glorified chloroform. Chloral hydrate enhances the GABA receptor complex, which can lead to both dependency and withdrawal and, more importantly, addiction. It is recommended to avoid in geriatric adults.

Meprobamate (marketed under the trade name Miltown®) was a best-selling anxiolytic drug before the advent of benzodiazepines. It is well known to have a high degree of physical dependence and is very sedating. It is recommended to avoid its use in geriatric adults.[35.]

The non-benzodiazepine hypnotics include the sleeping medications eszopiclone (Lunesta®), zolpidem (Ambien®) and zeleplon (Sonata®). They have long been known to cause serious side effects in the elderly, including delirium, falls, and fractures.[36.] Also, they have only minimal improvement in sleep latency and duration.[37] Chronic use of the medications can also lead to dependency, but short-term use has not. As a general rule, when medications increase delirium, falls, and fractures, they are best to be avoided in Geriatrics.

Ergot mesylates became famous for their ability to increase cerebral metabolism and blood flow. Their role was thought to improve outcomes in dementia, particularly vascular dementia. Controlled studies in patients with Alzheimer's disease found there was no advantage to the use of ergot mesylates compared to that of placebo; some studies suggest they may lower scores on some cognitive and behavioral rating scales. Further study is needed to determine the risk-benefit profile of ergot mesylates in the treatment of dementia, but there is no benefit to date in geriatric adults. Examples of trade names for this drug include Hydergine®, Hydergina®, Gerimal®, Niloric®, Redizork®, Alkergot®, Cicanol®, and Redergin®.

Table 6-10. The Endocrine System

Organ System or Therapeutic Category or Drug	Rationale	Recommendation	Quality/ Strength

Androgens
    methyltestosterone*
    testosterone*
	Potential for cardiac problem and contraindicated in men with prostate CA.	**Avoid** unless indicated for mod/severe hypogonadism.	Moderate / Weak

Desiccated thyroid	Concerns about cardiac effects; safer alternatives available.	**Avoid**	Low / Strong
Estrogens with or without progestins	Evidence of carcinogenic potential (breast and endometrium); lack of cardioprotective effect and cognitive protection in older women.	**Avoid** oral and topical patch; Topical vaginal cream is acceptable.	Oral and patch: strong Topical: weak
Growth hormone*	Effect on body composition is small and associated with edema, arthralgia, carpal tunnel syndrome, gynecomastia, impaired fasting glucose.	**Avoid** except as hormone replacement after pituitary gland removal.	High / Strong
Insulin, sliding scale	Higher risk of hypoglycemia without improvement in hyperglycemia management regardless of care setting.	**Avoid**	Moderate / Strong
Sulfonylureas (long duration) chlorpropamide	Chlorpropamide: prolonged half-life causing prolonged hypoglycemia; causes SIADH.	**Avoid**	High / Strong
glyburide*	Glyburide: greater risk of prolonged hypoglycemia in older adults.		

*New on 2012 American Geriatrics Society Updated Beers Criteria

(AGS Updated Beers Criteria for Potentially Inappropriate Medication Use in Older Adults (2012), www.americangeriatrics.org)

Androgens are a new category in Beers 2012, but certainly they are newsworthy items given the amount of controversy they have sparked in the last five years or so. Methyltestosterone and testosterone are the two that are listed. The rationale for their placement on the Beers Criteria is their potential for cardiac problems and their contraindication in men with prostate cancer (a risk that complements age). They also risk blood clots as is noted in the package insert.

Desiccated thyroid refers to porcine (or mixed beef and pork) thyroid that is prescribed for therapeutic use. It is commonly known as "Armour Thyroid." Geriatricians have long known there are safer alternatives available due to concerns about cardiac effects of desiccated thyroid. It should be pointed out that the quality of evidence is low, but the strength of the recommendation is strong.

Since the HERS[38] trial (the Heart Estrogen/Progestin Replacement Study) and the WHI[39] (Women's Health Initiative), estrogens with or without progestins are known to be risky in older adults due to the lack of cardioprotective effects that they were once touted to have. Additionally, the cardiogenic potential poses a significant risk. This risk applies to both the oral and patch forms of estrogen. The topical vaginal creams, however, pose less risk to patients, especially for the management of dypareunia and lower urinary tract symptoms (LUTS) and can be used without the same risk.

Growth hormone is also an addition to Beers 2012. Growth hormones are associated with risks like edema, generalized arthralgia, carpal tunnel syndrome, gynecomastia, and impaired fasting glucose levels. The quality of the evidence is high, and the strength of the recommendation is strong. It is recommended that it be avoided unless a patient has had a pituitary gland removal.

Sliding Scale Insulin (SSI), especially in the setting of long-term care, pose significant risks of hypoglycemia, which can be lethal for older adults. Some studies have even suggested that SSI should be avoided regardless of the care setting.[40] Individualizing plans are needed when older adults are diabetic, and frailty must be taken into consideration. This recommendation is strong due to the risk, and the quality of the evidence is moderate.

Additional anti-glycemic agents that should be avoided include the long-acting sulfonylureas since they increase the risk of hypoglycemia.[41] Two long-acting "secretagogues" are on Beers 2012. Chlorpropamide (Diabinese®) and glyburide (DiaBeta®; Micronase®) are known to have long half-lives—36 hours and 10 hours respectively—compared to glipizide (Glucotrol) which has a half-life of approximately 2.5 hours. As a consequence of the significant risks associated with hypoglycemia in the elderly, short-acting agents should be chosen if secretagogues are used.

Table 6-11. The Gastrointestinal System

Organ System or Therapeutic Category or Drug	Rationale	Recommendation	Quality/ Strength
Metoclopramide	Can cause extrapyramidal effects (EPS) including tardive dyskinesia; risk may be greater in frail older adults.	**Avoid**, unless for gastroparesis	Moderate / Strong
Mineral oil, oral*	Potential for aspiration and adverse effects; safer alternative available.	**Avoid**	Moderate / Strong
Trimethobenzamide	One of the least effective antiemetic drugs; can cause EPS	**Avoid**	High / Strong

*New on 2012 American Geriatrics Society Updated Beers Criteria

(AGS Updated Beers Criteria for Potentially Inappropriate Medication Use in Older Adults (2012), www.americangeriatrics.org)

Three medications made the Beers Criteria for the GI system. They include metoclopramide (Reglan®), oral mineral oils, and trimethobenzamide (Tigan®).

In reverse order, Tigan has long been known to be a relatively ineffective antiemetic,[42] but it can also cause extrapyramidal symptoms (EPS). The quality of the recommendation is high, and strength of the evidence is strong. If mineral oils are prescribed, they are prescribed for constipation. It is known as a lubricant laxative that works by keeping water in the stool and intestines. However, oral mineral oils have been known to potentiate aspiration, and safer alternatives are available for constipation.[43] Metoclopramide (Reglan®), an agent known to cause EPS and tardive dyskinesia,[44] should generally be avoided as a consequence of this risk. It has been prescribed for gastroesophageal reflux (GERD), vomiting, and symptoms of nausea, but the risk of EPS is high enough that it should be avoided for these circumstances if possible. The one consideration where Reglan may be an option is gastroparesis. However, even in this case, Reglan should be discontinued as soon as feasible.

The *majority* of analgesics (*see Tabele 6-12*) that pose a significant risk to older adults are NSAIDs. Non-Steroidal Anti-Inflammatory Drugs (including aspirin in doses greater than 325mg daily) markedly increase the risk of GI hemorrhage and peptic-ulcer disease (PUD). The highest risk groups are patients older than 75 years of age or those patients who use concomitant corticosteroids, anticoagulants, or anti-platelet agents.

Although proton-pump inhibitors (PPIs) or misoprostol reduces the risk of GI hemorrhage, it does not eliminate the risk. According to the Beers Criteria, upper GI ulcers, gross bleeding, or perforation by NSAIDs occurs in approximately 1% of patients treated for 3–6 months and 2–4% of patients for 1 year. These trends continue the longer the duration of NSAID use.

The recommendation is to avoid chronic use unless other alternatives are not effective. If a patient insists or must use NSAID therapy, then PPIs or misoprostol needs to be initiated at the same time to minimize their risk of GI hemorrhage.

The other two analgesic agents on the Beers Criteria include indomethacin (Indocin®) and ketorolac (Toradol®). Both of these agents increase the risk of GI hemorrhage and PUD. Additionally, indomethacin is associated with other adverse events which are primarily psychiatric in nature: agitation, anxiety, pseudodementia, psychosis, depression and hallucinations.[45]

Table 6-12. Analgesics

Organ System or Therapeutic Category or Drug	Rationale	Recommendation	Quality/ Strength
Non-COX-selective NSAIDs, oral ASA > 325mg/dl diclofenac* diflunisal* etodolac* fenoprofen* ibuprofen* ketoprofen* meclofenamate* mefenamic acid* meloxicam* nabumetone* naproxen oxaprozin piroxicam sulindac* tolmetin	Increases risk of GI bleeding and peptic ulcer disease (PUD) in high-risk groups, including those aged > 75 or taking orals or parenteral corticosteroids, anticoagulants, or antiplatelet agents. Use of PPI or misoprostol reduces but doesn't eliminate risk. Upper GI ulcers, gross bleeding or perforation by NSAIDs occur in approximately 1% of patients treated for 3-6 months and in approximately 2-4% of patients for 1 year. These trends continue with longer duration of use.	**Avoid** chronic use unless other altneratives are not effective and patient can take GI protective agent (PPI or misoprostol)	Moderate/ Strong
Indomethacin Ketorolac, including parenteral	Increases risk of GI hemor-rhage and PUD in high-risk groups. Of all the NSAIDs, indomethacin has the most adverse effects.	**Avoid**	Indomethacin: moderate Ketorolac: high / Strong
Meperidine*	Not an effective oral analgesic in dosages commonly used; may cause neurotoxicity; safer alternative available.	**Avoid**	High / Strong
Pentazocine	Opiod analgesic that causes CNS adverse effects, including confusion and hallucinations, more commonly than other narcotic drugs; is also a mixed agonist and antagonist; safer alternatives available.	**Avoid**	Low / Strong
Skeletal Muscle Relaxants carisoprodol chlorzoxazone cyclobenzaprine metaxaolone methocarbamol orphenadrine	Most muscle relaxants are poorly tolerated by older adults because of the anti-cholinergic adverse effects, sedation, risk of fracture; effectiveness at dosages tolerated by older adults is questionable.	**Avoid**	Moderate/ Strong

*New on 2012 American Geriatrics Society Updated Beers Criteria

(AGS Updated Beers Criteria for Potentially Inappropriate Medication Use in Older Adults (2012), www.americangeriatrics.org)

Meperidine (Demerol®) in the elderly has long been known to be potentially dangerous. The oral form of this agent has lower efficacy when weighed against comparable analgesics. More importantly, though, it may cause neurotoxicity which can lead to seizures.

Pentazocine (Talwin®) is an opioid analgesic that causes higher CNS adverse effects, including hallucinations and other psychomimetic effects, than do comparable analgesic agents. Since it is a mixed agonist and antagonist, efficacy varies. Quite simply, there are safer alternatives available. The recommendation is to avoid this agent; however, the quality of evidence is low with a strong recommendation.

Skeletal muscle relaxants are another agent commonly poorly tolerated by older adults because of the anticholinergic side effects. However, the agents listed in the Beers Criteria (Soma®, Parafon®, Flexeril® as examples) can also increase sedation and have been associated with an increased risk of fractures.[46] It is best to avoid these agents, but if they must be used, short-course treatment is preferred.

Inappropriate Medications due to Drug-Disease or Drug-Syndrome Interactions

Just as important as individual medications are to the Beers Criteria, so too are Drug-Disease Interactions or Drug-Syndrome Interactions. The table that follows (Table 6-13) lists some of the most common in Geriatric adults.

In heart failure, it is important to avoid drugs that promote fluid retention, which would thereby exacerbate heart failure. NSAIDs, including COX-2's, are included in the list. In addition, medications like diltiazem and verapamil are very important and potentially dangerous, especially in systolic heart failure, as they will promote and cause CHF. Pioglitizone (Actos®) traditionally used in diabetes, is another example of a medication that will promote fluid retention. Cilostazol (Pletal®) as well as dronedarone (Multaq®) are additional common examples of medications that can promote heart failure in Geriatrics.

Syncope is precisely defined as a transient loss of consciousness and postural tone characterized by rapid onset and short duration. The layman's term for this is fainting. Beers 2012 looked at several classes of medications that created a syncopal-type episode. The acetylcholinesterases (better known as the cognitive enhancers) are a class of medications that can and do result in syncope. Additionally, the peripheral alpha-blockers doxazosin, prazosin, and terazosin as well as nearly all of the tertiary TCAs are implicated in syncope.

In Geriatrics there are several medications affecting the Central Nervous System that lower the seizure threshold of a patient. Common medications that are overlooked but used in Geriatrics include buproprion (Wellbutrin®) and tramadol (Ultram®). Both of these medications lower the seizure threshold. It is best to avoid these medications in Geriatrics if an underlying seizure disorder exists.

Delirium is another common CNS side effect of many medications. As has been discussed, anticholinergic agents are probably the worst offenders. But so too are tricyclics, benzo's, corticosteroids, H2-antagonists, and sedative hypnotics. As was discussed earlier, delirium in the elderly can be lethal.

Additional CNS effects are under the heading dementia and cognitive impairment. It is always appropriate to attempt non-pharmacological approaches to care for these patients since medications such as anticholinergics agents, benzodiazepines like lorazepam and alprazolam, H2-antagonists, and sedative hypnotics can exacerbate a worsening of the memory. Furthermore, antipsychotics have long been associated with an increased risk of stroke and mortality in older adults with dementia. They should only be used as a last resort (both long-term and short-term).

Falls and fractures are very serious side effects of some medications. Those listed in Beers 2012 are duly noted for their adverse effects in causing falls: Anticonvulsants, antipsychotics, benzodiazepines, nonbenzodiazepines hypnotics, hypnotic agents like Ambien® and Lunesta®, as well as the tricyclic antidepressants, and all classes of the SSRIs. Medications like this should be reviewed should falls be frequent in older adults to determine if they are the cause.

Patients complaining of insomnia should have a medication review. Common medications that contribute to insomnia include any oral decongestants, stimulants, theophylline and caffeine. After this work-up has been done, then options for treatment can be explored.

Patients with Parkinson's disease should avoid medications that worsen their parkinsonian symptoms. All of the antipsychotics, except quetiapine and clozapine, worsen these symptoms. Additional agents that worsen these symptoms include metoclopramide, prochlorperazine, and promethazine.

When it comes to the gastrointestinal system, several agents should be considered problematic for older adults. Constipation is a ubiquitous example across the geriatric population where certain classes of medications should be avoided. These include oral anti-muscarinic agents for urinary incontinence, the nondihydropyridine calcium-channel blockers, first-generation antihistamines, and the anticholinergics and/or antispasmodic agents.

Another example includes those patients with a history of gastric or duodenal ulcers: Aspirin in doses greater than 325mg per day and the non-cox-2 selective NSAIDs risk exacerbating GI bleeding if used in the geriatric adult.

The final system to discuss involves the kidneys. Several discussions in the preceding chapters have noted the harm that many medications can do to the kidneys. In Stage IV and V chronic kidney disease (CKD), NSAIDs, and triamterene (alone or in combination) should be avoided since they may risk inducing renal failure.

For those women complaining of urinary incontinence, all estrogens (except vaginal estrogen) should be avoided since they can worsen the incontinence. Additionally, and usually in men, urinary incontinence can be worsened by any of the alpha-blockers, with more emphasis on doxazosin (Cardura®), prazosin (Minipress®), and terazosin (Hytrin®). On the other

Table 6-13. Medications Commonly Associated with Drug-Disease or Drug-Syndrome Interactions in Geriatric Adults

Disease or Syndrome	Drug	Rationale
Cardiovascular		

Heart Failure	NSAIDs and COX-2's
	Nondihydropyridine
	  CCBs in systolic heart failure
	  diltiazem
	  verapamil
	pioglitazone, rosiglitazone
	cilostazol
	dronedarone
		Potential to promote fluid retention and exacerbate heart failure.

Syncope	AChEI's
	Peripheral alpha blockers
	  doxazosin
	  prazosin
	  terazosin
	Tertiary TCAs
	  amitriptyline
	  clomipramine
	  doxepin
	  imipramine
	  trimipramine
	chlorpromazine, thiordazine and olanzapine
		Increases risk of orthostatic hypotension or bradycardia.

Central Nervous System		
Chronic seizures or epilepsy	buproprion chlorpromazine clozapine maprotiline olanzapine thioridazine thiothixene tramadol	Lowers seizure threshold; may be acceptable in patients with well-controlled seizures for whom alternative agents have not been effective.
Delirium	All TCAs Anticholinergic agents Benzodiazepines Chlorpromazine Corticosteroids H2-receptor antagonists meperidine Sedative hypnotics thioridazine	Worsens delirium in older adults; should taper if used chronically.
Dementia and Cognitive Impairment	Anticholinergic agents Benzodiazepines H2-receptor antagonists zolpidem Antipsychotics, chronic and PRN use	Avoid due to the adverse CNS effects. Avoid antipsychotics for behavioral problems of dementia unless options have failed, and patient is a threat to self or others. Antipsychotics are associated with an increased risk of cerebrovascular accident (stroke) and mortality in older adults with dementia

(Continued).

73

Table 6-13 (continued). Medications Commonly Associated with Drug-Disease or Drug-Syndrome Interactions in Geriatric Adults

Disease or Syndrome	Drug	Rationale
Central Nervous System (continued)		

History of falls and fractures	Anticonvulsants
	Antipsychotics
	Benzodiazepines
	Nonbenzodiazepine hypnotics
	  eszopiclone
	  zaleplon
	  zolpidem
	TCAs and SSRIs
		Ability to produce ataxia, impaired psychomotor function, syncope, and additional falls; shorter-acting benzodiazepines are not safer than long-acting ones

Insomnia	Oral decongestants
	  psuedophedrine
	  phenylephrine
	Stimulants
	  amphetamine
	  methylphenidate
	  pemoline
	Theobromines
	  theophylline
	  Caffeine
		CNS stimulants effects

Parkinson's disease	All antipsychotics (except quetiapine and clozapine)
	Antiemetics
	  metoclopramide
	  prochlorperazine
	  promethazine
		Dopamine receptor antagonists with potential to worsen parkinsonian symptoms. Quetiapine and clozapine appear to be less likely to precipitate worsening of Parkinson's

(Continued)

(Continued)

Disease or Syndrome	Drug	Rationale
Gastrointestinal		

Chronic Constipation	Oral antimuscarines for urinary incontinence
	  darifenacin
	  fesoterodine
	  oxybutynin (oral)
	  solifenacin
	  tolterodine
	  trospium
	Nondihydropyridine CCBs
	  diltiazem
	  verapamil
	First-generation antihistamines as single agent or part of combination products
	  brompheniramine (various)
	  carbinoxamine
	  chlorpheniramine
	  clemastine (various)
	  cyproheptadine
	  dexbrompheniramine
	  dexchlorpheniramine (various)
	  diphenhydramine
	  doxylamine
	  hydroxyzine
	  promethazine
	  triprolidine
	Anticholinergics and Antispasmodics
	  antipsychtoics
	  belladona alkaloids
	  clidinium-chlordiazepoxide
	  dicyclomine
	  hyoscyamine
	  propantheline
	  scopalamine
	  tertiary TCAs
	    amitriptyline
	    clomipramine
	    doxepin
	    imipramine
	    trimipramine	

History of gastric or duodenal ulcers	ASA (>325mg/d) Non-COX-2 selective NSAIDs	May exacerbate existing ulcers or cause new or additional ulcers
Kidney and Urinary Tract		
Chronic kidney diseases Stages IV and V	NSAIDs triamterene (alone or in combination)	May increase risk of kidney injury
Urinary incontinence (all types in women)	Estrogen (oral or transdermal ONLY)	Aggravation of incontinence
Lower urinary tract symptoms or BPH	Inhaled anticholinergic agents Strongly anticholinergic drugs, except antimuscarinic drugs for urinary incontinence	

Stress or mixed urinary incontinence	Alpha Blockers
	  doxazosin
	  prazosin
	  terazosin
		Aggravation of incontinence

(AGS Updated Beers Criteria for Potentially Inappropriate Medication Use in Older Adults (2012), www.americangeriatrics.org)

Chapter 7
STOPP and START

STOPP (Screening Tool of Older Persons' Prescriptions) and START (Screening Tool to Alert to Right Treatment) were formulated to identify potentially inappropriate medications and potential errors of omissions in older patients.[47]

The concept of STOPP and START was originally designed to counteract some of the flaws of the original Beers list. To some degree Beers 2012 emulated STOPP and START, but the ease of using and "sifting" through STOPP and START has made it a tool that is, frankly, simpler to use and to understand.

STOPP is comprised of 65 clinically significant criteria for potentially inappropriate prescribing in older people. Each criterion is accompanied by a concise explanation of why the drug is there. START consists of 22 evidence-based prescribing indicators for commonly encountered diseases in older people.

The 18-member expert panel from academic centers in Ireland and the United Kingdom created STOPP and START to capture common and important instances of inappropriate prescribing, and organized it by physiological systems. They also paid special attention to drugs affecting fall risk and opiate use in elders. Finally, they included medications that improve outcomes and quality of life as well. It was a unique and appropriate way to determine medications to be either discontinued or safely used in geriatric adults.

STOPP and the Cardiovascular System
- Digoxin at a long-term dose > 125mcg/day with impaired renal function.
- Loop diuretic for dependent ankle edema without any clinical signs of heart failure.
  - no evidence of efficacy, compression hose usually more appropriate

- Loop diuretic as first-line monotherapy for hypertension
- Thiazide diuretic with a history of gout as it is likely to exacerbate the gout.
- Non-cardioselective beta-blocker (BB) with chronic obstructive pulmonary disease (COPD) due to risk of bronchospasm.
- Use of a beta-blocker in combination with verapamil as it may cause heart block.
- Use of diltiazem or verapamil with NYHA Class III or IV heart failure as it may worsen heart failure.
- Use of calcium channel blockers (CCB) with chronic constipation since it may exacerbate constipation.
- Aspirin with a past history of peptic ulcer disease without histamine H2-receptor antagonist or proton-pump inhibitor (increases risks of bleeding).
- Aspirin with no history of coronary, cerebral or peripheral arterial symptoms or occlusive arterial event (not indicated).
- Warfarin for first, uncomplicated deep venous thrombosis for longer than 6 months duration; there is no proven added benefit.
- Warfarin for first uncomplicated pulmonary embolus for longer than 12 months duration; there is no proven added benefit.

In general, medications with narrow therapeutic ranges should be used cautiously in older adults since renal function tends to affect the outcomes of these medications. Digoxin is one such medication and is also listed in the Beers Criteria. In older adults, digoxin doses greater than 125mcg (.125mg) risk toxicity. This is of particular importance in the presence of renal insufficiency or an Acute Kidney Injury (AKI) occurring when older adults become dehydrated. As was stated in Chapter 6, should a patient be taking doses of digoxin greater than 125mcg, a cardiologist should support its use.

Loop diuretics increase risks of dehydration for any patient, but in the old and frail, this is of particular importance. Loop diuretics used for dependent ankle edema without any clinical signs of failure has not been proven efficacious, but has been shown to increase the risk of an acute kidney injury. In addition, loop diuretics should not be used as first-line monotherapy for hypertension.

Thiazide diuretics (hydrochlorothiazide, chlorthalidone) have long been known to exacerbate gout and should be avoided in patients with this history.

All practitioners learn about the risks associated with using beta-blockers in patients with a history of Chronic Obstructive Pulmonary Disease (COPD). There is a risk of bronchospasm associated with their use; however, COPD was associated with a 3.5-fold increase in the rate of Acute Myocardial Infarction (AMI) compared to those with no COPD.[48] Consequently, beta-blockers (BB) are indeed *appropriate* for patients with COPD; however, practitioners should use selective beta-blockers (nebivolol, metoprolol) rather than non-selective beta-blockers (carvedilol, propranolol) due to the risk of bronchospasm.

Any beta-blocker used in combination with verapamil can cause a complete heart block and therefore should be avoided in combination.

In addition, calcium channel blockers (CCBs) are well known to worsen constipation. As a general rule, when calcium channel blockers are initiated, patients may benefit from medications that prevent constipation.

Aspirin inherently increases the risk of GI hemorrhage, especially as the dose is increased or if it is used in the presence of other NSAIDs.[49] If a patient *has a history* of peptic ulcer disease (PUD) and is on aspirin, then an H2-antagonist or proton-pump inhibitor (PPI) should be prescribed concomitantly for safety.

Evidence has now shown that in the absence of coronary, cerebral, or peripheral arterial disease or symptoms thereof, aspirin is no longer a needed preventative measure. Primary prevention with the use of aspirin has not shown benefit in the latest studies.[50] An individual's potential clinical benefit from aspirin depends on his or her baseline risk, which can be determined by using the Clinician Fact Sheet from the U.S. Preventive Task Force.[51] (See *START and the Endocrine System for exceptions*).

Warfarin also carries with it significant risks. Given the risk of gastrointestinal hemorrhage (1.1% per year) and intracranial hemorrhage (.8% per year), it should be discontinued WHEN appropriate. Warfarin for a *first*, uncomplicated deep venous thrombosis (DVT) for longer than 6 months of duration is no longer warranted because the risk of a life-threatening hemorrhage outweighs the benefit it provides. Furthermore, warfarin for a *first* uncomplicated pulmonary embolus for longer than 12 months duration is not warranted and should be discontinued as well.

STOPP and the Central Nervous System
- Tricyclic antidepressants (TCA's) with dementia (risk of worsening cognitive impairment).
- TCA's with glaucoma (likely to exacerbate glaucoma).
- TCA's with cardiac conductive abnormalities (pro-arrhythmic effects).
- TCA's with constipation (likely to worsen constipation).
- TCA's with an opiate or calcium channel blocker (risk of severe constipation).
- TCA's with prostatism or prior history of urinary retention (risk of urinary retention).
- Long-term (i.e. >1 month), long-acting benzodiazepines, e.g., chlordiazepoxide and benzodiazepines with long-acting metabolites, e.g., diazepam (risk of prolonged sedation, confusion, impaired balance, falls).
- Long-term first-generation neuroleptics (>1 month) in those with parkinsonism (likely to worsen extrapyramidal symptoms).
- Phenothiazines in patients with epilepsy (may lower seizure threshold).

- Selective serotonin re-uptake inhibitors (SSRI's) with a history of clinically significant hyponatremia (non-iatrogenic hyponatremia < 130 mmol/L within the previous 2 months).
- Prolonged use (>1 week) of first generation antihistamines, i.e., diphenhydramine, chlorpheniramine, promethazine (risk of sedation and anticholinergic side effects).

As mentioned earlier (*see Chapter 6*), tricyclic antidepressants (TCA's) are risky when used in geriatric adults. They are strongly anti-cholinergic medications and therefore are known to cause cardiac conduction abnormalities. They will also worsen cognition, symptoms associated with glaucoma, constipation (especially if used in the presence of a opiate or calcium channel blocker), and urinary retention.

There is little place for the use of long-term benzodiazepines (chlordiazepoxide - Librium; diazepam - Valium) due to the marked risk of prolonged sedation, impaired balance, and falls. As a general rule, when falls are listed as a side effect of any medication, their use should be reconsidered for the elderly. Long-acting benzodiazepines are also known to be habit-forming and for that reason, should be avoided in geriatrics.

Long-term first-generation neuroleptics also known as "typical" antipsychotics comprise drugs like haloperidol (Haldol®), thioridazine (Mellaril®), fluphenazine (Prolixin®), and chlorpromazine (Thorazine®) to name a few. The risk of extrapyramidal symptoms (EPS) is known to be very high with these agents. They are not recommended in geriatrics except in palliative or hospice care.

Phenothiazines range a broad spectrum of medications; however, some of the most common are also commonly used in geriatric adults despite their risk of lowering the seizure threshold. Examples include prochlorperazine (Compazine®) and promethazine (Phenergan®).

Other psychotropic agents that were included in STOPP, despite quite frequent use in geriatrics, include the selective serotonin reuptake inhibitors (SSRIs) which have a clinical risk of causing hyponatremia. The reported incidence of SSRI-associated hyponatremia has been variable, ranging from 0.5 to 32 percent, and was most often observed in older adults [52]. STOPP recommends not initiating SSRIs (this also includes SNRIs) for serum sodium of less than 130mmol/L within the previous *two months*. This recommendation is due to the risk of causing clinically significant hyponatremia, which can lead to seizures.

STOPP and the Gastrointestinal System

- Diphenoxylate, loperamide or codeine phosphate for treatment of diarrhea of unknown cause (risk of delayed diagnosis, may exacerbate constipation with overflow diarrhea, may precipitate toxic megacolon in inflammatory bowel disease, and may delay recovery in unrecognized gastroenteritis).
- Diphenoxylate, loperamide or codeine phosphate for treatment of severe infective gastroenteritis, i.e., bloody diarrhea, high fever, or severe systemic toxicity (risk of exacerbation or sepsis).
- Prochlorperazine or metoclopramide with Parkinsonism (risk of exacerbating Parkinsonism).
- PPI for peptic ulcer disease for longer than > 8 weeks in patients that are asymptomatic (not indicated).
- Anticholinergic antispasmodic drugs with chronic constipation, e.g., dicyclomine (risk of exacerbation of constipation).

Diphenoxylate (Lomotil®), loperamide (Imodium®) or codeine phosphate (discontinued in the United States) for treatment of diarrhea of unknown cause is risky, especially in older adults. Using these agents, even as needed or PRN, can delay the true diagnosis of the cause of diarrhea and may exacerbate constipation in patients who are already at risk of constipation. The greatest risk of these agents is that it may precipitate a toxic megacolon, which, as many know, can lead to systemic toxicity or septicemia. They are not recommended in geriatric adults.

Furthermore, prochlorperazine (Compazine®) or metoclopramide (Reglan®) with Parkinson's Disease or Parkinsonisms may exacerbate these symptoms.

The use of proton-pump inhibitors for peptic ulcer disease (PUD) is a mainstay treatment. However, treatment longer than 8 weeks in patients that are asymptomatic is typically not indicated.

Anticholinergic antispasmodics should be avoided in geriatric adults due to the risk of exacerbating constipation. Examples of these agents include hyoscyamine (Anaspaz®), belladona alkaloids (Donnatal®), dicyclomine (Bentyl®) and scopolamine (Scopace®).

STOPP and the Respiratory System
- Theophylline as monotherapy for COPD (there are safer, more effective alternatives; risk of adverse effects due to narrow therapeutic index).
- Systemic corticosteroids instead of inhaled corticosteroids for maintenance therapy in moderate-severe COPD (unnecessary exposure to long-term side effects of systemic steroids).
- Nebulized ipratropium with glaucoma (may exacerbate glaucoma).

Theophylline as a monotherapy for COPD is not indicated, especially considering there are more effective alternatives available. In addition, and as has been stated before, any medication that has a narrow therapeutic window must be used cautiously in older adults.

Inhaled corticosteroids are preferred agents over systemic corticosteroids in moderate-severe COPD. The long-term side effects of systemic steroids include GI hemorrhage, diabetes mellitus, glaucoma, osteoporosis, edema and hypertension.

Narrow angle glaucoma (a serious eye condition that may cause loss of vision), may worsen and become an acute end-angle glaucoma with the use of nebulized ipratropium. It should be noted this does not apply to inhaled tiotropium.

STOPP and the Musculoskeletal System

- Non-steroidal anti-inflammatory drugs (NSAIDs) with history of peptic ulcer disease or gastrointestinal bleeding, unless with concurrent histamine H2-receptor antagonist or PPI (risk of peptic ulcer relapse).
- NSAIDs with moderate-severe hypertension (risk of exacerbation of hypertension.)
- NSAIDs with heart failure (risk of exacerbation of heart failure).
- Long-term use of NSAIDs (>3 months) for relief of mild joint pain in osteoarthritis (simple analgesics preferable and usually as effective for pain relief).
- Warfarin and NSAIDs together (risk of gastrointestinal bleeding).
- NSAIDs with chronic renal failure/CKD III (risk of deterioration in renal function).
- Long-term corticosteroids (>3 months) as monotherapy for rheumatoid arthritis or osteoarthritis (risk of major systemic corticosteroid side effects).
- Long-term NSAIDs or colchicine for chronic treatment of gout where there is no contraindication to allopurinol (allopurinol is the first choice prophylactic drug in gout).

The risks associated with non-steroidal, anti-inflammatory drugs (NSAIDs) in older adults have long been known and have been discussed in detail in Chapters 3–5.

Only in rare cases will older adults require them to manage pain. In the rare occasion an older adult does require NSAIDs, concurrent H2-antagonists or proton-pump inhibitors (PPIs) should be prescribed to protect against future GI hemorrhage.

Furthermore, NSAIDs in the presence of moderate-severe hypertension or heart failure, for those with Chronic Kidney Disease (CKD) Stage III (*Note: Beers Criteria suggests avoiding NSAIDs for CKD IV or V*), and for those taking warfarin, should be avoided. Although NSAIDs are warranted for short-term relief of pain in the treatment of gout, long-term management is not indicated unless there is a contraindication to allopurinol.

The World Health Organization (WHO) has an analgesic ladder that is usually preferred in geriatrics to NSAIDs for pain relief.[53] When possible, practitioners should attempt to follow the analgesic ladder for pain relief.

Finally, a handful of patients may use systemic corticosteroids as monotherapy for either rheumatoid arthritis or, less commonly, osteoarthritis. Prolonged use of these agents poses risks (*see STOPP and the Respiratory System*); consequently, alternate agents or specialty referral should be considered.

STOPP and the Urogenital System
- Bladder antimuscarinic drugs with dementia (risk of increased confusion, agitation).
- Bladder antimuscarinic drugs with chronic glaucoma (risk of acute exacerbation of glaucoma).
- Bladder antimuscarinic drugs with chronic constipation (risk of exacerbation of constipation).
- Bladder antimuscarinic drugs with chronic prostatism (risk of urinary retention).
- Alpha-blockers in males with frequent incontinence, i.e., one or more episodes of daily incontinence (risk of urinary frequency and worsening of incontinence).
- Alpha-blockers with long-term urinary catheter *in situ*, i.e., more than 2 months (drug not indicated).

Bladder antimuscarinic drugs include a large class of medications that induce delirium (worsen dementia) and behaviors associated with dementia, risk acute exacerbation of glaucoma, worsen constipation, and increase the likelihood of urinary retention. Agents in this class include tolterodine (Detrol or Detrol LA®), oxybutinin (Ditropan, Ditropan XL, Oxytrol®), darifenacin (Enablex®), trospium (Sanctura or Sanctura XR®), fesoterodine (Toviaz®), flavoxate (Urispas®) and solifenacin (Vesicare®). Do not be fooled into believing that the newer agents are less risky for any of the above side effects. All of these medications carry these risks.

STOPP and the Endocrine System
- Chlorpropamide with type-2 diabetes mellitus (risk of prolonged hypoglycemia).
- Beta-blockers in those with diabetes mellitus and frequent hypoglycemic episodes, i.e., **One** episode per month (risk of masking hypoglycemic symptoms).
- Estrogens with a history of breast cancer or venous thromboembolism (increased risk of recurrence).
- Estrogens without progesterone in patients with intact uterus (risk of endometrial cancer).

Chlorpropamide (Diabinese®) is a secretagogue. It stimulates pancreatic islet beta cells to release insulin. The half-life of this medication is approximately 36 hours. These islet cells are indifferent to producing insulin even when an older adult stops eating or has nausea leading to anorexia or diarrhea or vomiting. Consequently, the risk of hypoglycemia is increased and enhanced with long-acting agents like chlorpropamide.

Beta-blockers, when used in diabetics, may lead to a decreased risk of myocardial infarction. However, for those patients who are "brittle" and whose sugars rise and fall very quickly, beta-blockers have been known to "mask" hypoglycemia and consequently lead to the risk of an adverse drug event. Patients who have greater than or equal to one episode of hypoglycemia in the presence of a beta-blocker should have the beta-blocker discontinued.

The Women's Health Initiative and the HERS trials demonstrated the risk of prolonged use of estrogens *(see Chapter 6)*. Estrogen alone with a history of breast cancer or venous thromboembolism (VTE) carries a risk of recurrence. Likewise, estrogens without progesterone in patients with an intact uterus risk endometrial cancer.

STOPP those Drugs that Increase the Risk of Falls
- Benzodiazepines (sedative, may cause reduced sensorium, impair balance).
- Neuroleptic drugs (may cause gait dyspraxia or Parkinsonism).
- First-generation antihistamines (sedative, may impair sensorium).
- Vasodilator drugs known to cause hypotension in those with persistent postural hypotension, i.e., recurrent > 20mmHg drop in systolic blood pressure, i.e., alpha-2-adrenergic stimulators (centrally-acting antihypertensives) or alpha-1-antagonists or (risk of syncope, falls).
- Long-term opiates in those with recurrent falls (risk of drowsiness, postural hypotension, vertigo).

Whenever the words *fall* or *fracture* appear in the same sentence as the word *geriatric*, the practitioner must consider the medication being prescribed or used. Benzodiazepines, neuroleptics agents, and first-generation anti-histamines are some of the most common medications that can lead to falls and subsequent fractures. Additionally, vasodilator drugs such as alpha-2-adrenergic stimulators (clonidine) and alpha-1-antagonists (doxazosin) contribute to falls. Lastly, except in the presence of those on hospice or palliative care, long-term opiates in patients with recurrent falls should be discontinued. Short-term opioids, on the other hand, can and should be considered.

STOPP and Analgesics

- Use of long-term powerful opiates, e.g., morphine or fentanyl, as first-line therapy for mild-moderate pain (WHO analgesic ladder not observed).
- Regular opiates for more than 2 weeks in those with chronic constipation without concurrent use of laxatives (risk of severe constipation).
- Long-term opiates in those with dementia unless indicted for palliative care or management of moderate/severe chronic pain syndrome (risk of exacerbation of cognitive impairment).

When it comes to pain, the World Health Organization follows an "analgesic ladder" that is very specific. Use of this ladder should be considered. Pain medications that are titrated appropriately in older adults risk lethargy, fatigue, constipation, and delirium.

START (Screening Tool to Alert to Right Treatment)

The biggest advantage of STOPP and START is the Screening Tool to Alert to Right Treatment. It has been rare in Geriatrics to find instances where practitioners evaluate how to improve both quality and quantity of life, but START has accomplished that.

START and the Cardiovascular System

- Warfarin in the presence of chronic atrial fibrillation.
- Aspirin in the presence of chronic atrial fibrillation where warfarin, but not aspirin, is contra-indicated.
- Aspirin with a documented history of coronary artery disease/cerebrovascular disease, or aspirin OR clopidogrel in the presence of peripheral vascular disease in patients with sinus rhythm.
- Antihypertensive therapy where systolic blood pressure consistently >150 mmHg unless symptomatic below this range.

- Statin therapy with a documented history of coronary, cerebral or peripheral vascular disease, where the patient's functional status remains independent for activities of daily living, and life expectancy is >5 years.
- Angiotensin converting enzyme (ACE) inhibitor with chronic heart failure.
- ACE inhibitor following acute myocardial infarction.
- Beta-blocker with chronic stable angina.

Despite the risks associated with warfarin, it is still the standard of care for atrial fibrillation; the risk of stroke, in most circumstances can outweigh the risk associated with warfarin use. Where warfarin is contraindicated, however, low-dose aspirin is an acceptable choice.

Aspirin too, is indicated for those with a documented history of coronary artery disease (CAD), cerebrovascular disease (CVD) or aspirin or clopidogrel (Plavix®) in the presence of peripheral vascular disease (PVD).

When systolic blood pressures are greater than 150 mmHg, treatment should be considered. The American Geriatrics Society recommends treatment to standards of the JNC-VII, unless when blood pressures run low in older adults, or older adults are symptomatic (dizzy or lightheaded). Unlike JNC-VII guidelines, START recommended treatment levels to a different standard due to the risk of falls associated with having too low of a blood pressure.

Statins are medications that have substantial efficacy, and they should be used with a documented history of coronary, cerebral, or peripheral vascular disease. However, statins are best used when the patient's functional status remains independent for activities of daily living, and life expectancy is greater than 5 years. Otherwise, statins may not be necessary for older adults.

Angiotensin converting enzyme (ACE) inhibitors have many benefits in older adults. Some of the distinct advantages include benefits for heart failure and myocardial infarction. Beta-blockers make the START criteria for patients with chronic stable angina.

START and the Respiratory System
• Regular inhaled beta-2 agonist or inhaled anticholinergic agent for mild to moderate asthma or COPD.
• Regular inhaled corticosteroid for moderate-severe asthma or COPD as defined by the WHO.
• Continuous oxygen with documented chronic hypoxia.

Patients with mild-to-moderate COPD or asthma should START beta-2-agonists or inhaled anticholinergic agents. Additionally, inhaled (not to be confused with oral) corticosteroids for moderate-to-severe asthma or COPD as defined by the World Health Organization and GOLD standards should be STARTed in older adults. Finally, for those older patients who are hypoxic, the practitioner should START oxygen as it has been shown to improve outcomes data for older adults but also for their quality of life.

START and the Central Nervous System
• L-DOPA in idiopathic Parkinson's disease with definite functional impairment and resultant disability without orthostatic hypotension.
• Antidepressant drug in the presence of moderate-severe depressive symptoms lasting at least two months.

Two medications make the START criteria in the Central Nervous System. The first is L-Dopa for patients with Parkinson's Disease in the absence of orthostatic hypotension. The second agents are anti-depressants in the presence of moderate-to-severe depression.

START and the Gastrointestinal System
• Proton-pump inhibitor with severe GERD or peptic strictures requiring dilatation.
• Fiber supplement for chronic, symptomatic diverticular disease with constipation.

In the GI system, the use of PPIs with severe reflux or peptic strictures requiring dilatation SHOULD be utilized and continued. For practical purposes, START also recommends fiber supplementation for those patients with chronic, symptomatic diverticular disease in the presence of constipation.

START and the Musculoskeletal System
• Disease-modifying anti-rheumatic drugs (DMARDs) with active moderate-severe rheumatoid disease lasting >12 weeks.
• Bisphosphonates in patients taking maintenance oral corticosteroid therapy unless GFR < 50mL/min.
• Calcium and vitamin D supplement in patients with known osteopenia/osteoporosis or any women who are postmenopausal.

The musculoskeletal system is widely affected in geriatric patients. It is therefore recommended that, for patients with moderate-to-severe rheumatoid disease, DMARDs (disease-modifying anti-rheumatic drugs) be initiated. It is best to do this with the guidance of a rheumatologist.

Bisphosphonates should also be considered in older adults using oral corticosteroids. This recommendation is given for older adults if their GFR is >50mL/min/1.73m^2.

Finally, calcium and vitamin D supplementation is recommended in any postmenopausal women or those with known osteopenia or osteoporosis.

START and the Endocrine System

- Metformin with type 2 diabetes±metabolic syndrome (unless GFR < 50mL/min)
- ACE inhibitor or angiotensin receptor blocker in diabetes with nephropathy, i.e., overt urinalysis proteinuria or microalbuminuria
- Antiplatelet therapy in diabetes mellitus if one or more co-existing major cardiovascular risk factors are present (hypertension, hypercholesterolemia, smoking history)
- Statin therapy in diabetes mellitus if one or more co-existing major cardiovascular risk factor present

Metformin (Glucophage) is one of those medications that really has stood the test of time. Some of the most impressive studies for its use come from the United Kingdom Prospective Diabetes Study (UKPDS). START recommends its use for patients with type II diabetes or for those patients with metabolic syndrome. Two contraindications should be considered, however, when prescribing metformin. As was discussed earlier, metformin should not be used in female patients with a serum creatinine of 1.4 or greater and in men with a serum creatinine of 1.5 or greater. Additionally, if the GFR is less than $50mL/min/1.73m^2$, it should be avoided.

In the endocrine system, ACE inhibitors or angiotensin receptor blockers (ARBs) are medications that provide benefit in diabetes with nephropathy. Additionally, in patients who are diabetic, providers should START antiplatelet therapy if one or more co-existing major cardiovascular risk factors are present such as hypertension, hypercholesterolemia, or smoking history. Lastly, the statins play a significant role, as well, in diabetes in the presence of those same major cardiovascular risk factors. The exclusion that was discussed in STOPP hold true however. When the patient's functional status lacks independence and the life expectancy is <5 years, their use should be questioned.

Chapter 8
Practical Guidelines for Prescribers

As a general rule, inappropriate prescribing starts by using drug doses that are too high for elderly populations. In the United States, most studies just are not done on the elderly; consequently, practitioners may start older adults on medication doses that would just not be appropriate for them. Furthermore, especially when speaking about the "old, old" (85 years or older), high medication doses can really be dangerous.

The list that follows includes practical guidelines for safe prescribing in the elderly adult:

- Consider non-pharmacological agents for treatment.
- Avoid prescribing prior to having a high "index of suspicion" for a diagnosis.
- Start "low" and "go slow."
- Document the indication for each new drug that is started (to avoid using unnecessary drugs and to serve as a reminder of why the drug was chosen).
- Adjust doses for renal and hepatic impairment in the elderly.
- Avoid initiating two agents at the same time.
- Reach "target" dose before switching or adding additional agents (understand $t_{1/2}$).
- Document the risk of therapy versus its benefit.
- Choose the safest possible alternative (e.g., choose Tylenol for arthritis over an NSAID).
- Check for potential drug-disease and drug-drug interactions.
- Avoid the "prescribing cascade" by first determining if any new symptom(s) are the consequence of an existing drug.
- Attempt to prescribe a drug that will treat more than one existing problem (Remeron may be used for both depression and to stimulate appetite).

- Determine therapeutic endpoints and, most important, document them. If a therapeutic endpoint is not achieved because the drug either has a side effect or just is not working, discontinue the medication.
- Explain why the drug is being taken and educate patients about common adverse effects of each drug.

As noted above, doses of medications in older adults should be lower than those of their young counterparts. Starting doses of about one third to one half the usual non-geriatric adult dose is recommended. Once the drug is shown to be working, it can be followed by upward titration, when and where appropriate, until there is a desired effect. Up-titration frequency is dictated by a concrete understanding of a medication's half-life and a patient's renal clearance. Since steady-state is not achieved for 5 to 6 half-lives, practitioners should evaluate for adverse effects before adjusting dosage or frequency of administration.

It is particularly important to reconsider medication appropriateness and, more importantly, to continually evaluate it at subsequent visits. A model for appropriate prescribing for older patients is shown in Table 8-1. The process considers a life expectancy and quality-of-life measures in reviewing the need for existing medications and in making new prescribing decisions. For example, if a patient's life expectancy is short, and the goals of care are more palliative in approach, then prescribing a medication to prevent heart disease, which requires several years to realize any benefit, may not be considered appropriate. This is most evident when patients have severe dementia.[54]

Table 8-1. Appropriate Prescribing in the Elderly[55]

1. Is there an indication for the drug?
2. Is the medication effective for the condition?
3. Is the dosage correct?
4. Are the directions correct?
5. Are the directions practical?
6. Are there clinically significant drug-drug Interactions?
7. Are there clinically significant drug-disease/condition interactions?
8. Is there unnecessary duplication with other drugs?
9. Is the duration of therapy acceptable?
10. Is this drug the least expensive alternative compared with others of equal usefulness?

Much attention has been paid to overprescribing for older adults. As an example, a patient with a diabetes might be recommended to be on an anti-glycemic agent (or two), beta-blocker, ACE inhibitor, aspirin, and statin. In this context, the risk for a drug-drug interaction doubles if one additional medication would be added *(see Chapter 4)*. On the other hand, under-prescribing appropriate medications is also of concern. One study of older adults in a VA outpatient population with a mean age of 75 years documented underuse of appropriate medications as many as 64 percent of the time.[51] Despite this, it should be pointed out that "under-prescribing" also might be prevalent as a way to improve compliance with essential medications while limiting drug interactions to minimize risk and improve quality of life.

A Stepwise Approach to Prescribing
When it is deemed necessary to prescribe, practitioners should follow certain steps and abide by certain guidelines:

1. Review and re-review current drug therapy
Periodic but continual evaluation of a patient's drug regimen is an essential component in caring for the elderly. As such, a review of medications (annually for clinic patients and once every three months for patients in Assisted Living Facilities and Long-Term Care) may result in positive changes to or even discontinuation of prescribed drug therapy. Changes may include discontinuing a therapy (as needed or routine) prescribed for either an acute situation or an indication that no longer exists. It may also include substituting a therapy with a potentially safer agent, a change in drug dosage, or a new more appropriate medication. Medication reviews should consider whether an acute or chronic change in patient condition might necessitate dosing adjustment, determine if there is a potential for a drug-drug interaction, reflect a drug side effect, or decide whether the current drug regimen could be decreased.

Furthermore, at least once annually (or after ANY hospitalization), encourage patients to bring all (*everything*) of the bottles or pills they are using or *have used* in the past year; it is best to ask them to empty their medicine cabinet and bring those medications in. Patients may not consider over-the-counter products, ointments, vitamins, eye drops, or herbal medicines to be drug therapies. Make sure the practitioner mentions that the visit will be only to review medications and nothing else.

2. Discontinue unnecessary therapy

Appropriately, clinicians may feel reluctant to stop certain medications, especially if the patient seems to be tolerating the therapy and the treatment was not initiated by the clinician reviewing the patient. A common example is digoxin, which has many drug-drug interactions, risks digoxin toxicity, and has variable efficacy in older adults. However, it also has benefits in heart failure and atrial fibrillation.

The decision to discontinue a medication is determined in part by the goals of care for that patient and the risks of adverse effects for that patient. One approach to assessing whether a drug is truly necessary for a given patient is presented in Chapter 9. Furthermore, some preventive and other therapies may no longer be beneficial to patients with shorter-than-expected life spans.

It is reasonable to taper off most medications so as to minimize withdrawal reactions and to allow symptom monitoring, unless dangerous signs or symptoms indicate a need for abrupt medication withdrawal. Certain common drugs require tapering, including beta-blockers, opioids, barbiturates, clonidine, gabapentin, and antidepressants. In general, the appropriateness of any therapy should be reconsidered when other medical conditions develop that impact a patient's long-term prognosis, unless the therapies are thought to increase comfort or the patient and/or family desire it.

3. Consider adverse drug events for any new symptom

Before adding any new therapy to the patient's drug regimen, carefully consider whether a new medical condition could be linked to an existing drug therapy. Clinicians should evaluate the drug regimen approximately 2 months prior to see if the symptom may be related to the drug therapy. Doing so could avoid a prescribing cascade.

4. ALWAYS consider non-pharmacologic approaches

Some conditions in older adults may benefit from simple lifestyle modification in lieu of pharmacotherapy. As an example, simple weight loss and reduced sodium intake, as shown in the Trial of Non-pharmacologic Interventions in the Elderly (TONE trial), allowed for discontinuation of antihypertensive medication in about 40 percent of the cases.[57]

5. Substitute with safer alternatives

When drug therapy is indicated for the older patient, it may be possible to substitute a safer alternative for the current regimen. As an example, the newer seizure agents (Lamictal® or Keppra®) have fewer drug-drug interactions and do not require blood monitoring. In addition, as older adults become "older" they may not need the same doses of medications they required as "younger" older adults.

6. Reduce the dose

Many adverse drug events are dose-related. When prescribing drug therapies, it is important to use the lowest dose needed to obtain a clinical benefit.

7. Simplify the dosing schedule

When multiple medications are taken, the complexity around them increases the likelihood of poor compliance or confusion with dosing. Studies indicate that once-daily medical regimens result in up to twice as many adherent days.[58]

Chapter 9

An Algorithm to Discontinuing Medications

  The Garfinkel Method (Figure 9-1), is an algorithm designed to feasibly and safely discontinue medications and address the issue of polypharmacy in the elderly.[59] As is seen in the algorithm, the practitioner starts by determining if an evidence-based consensus exists for the use of, and continuation of, the medication in question. If the practitioner can determine that the medication in question is indicated at its current dose, considering the patient's age group and disability level, and that the benefits outweigh the risk, then the medication should be continued. Otherwise, the practitioner should move to the next step in the algorithm.

  This next step is to determine if the indication is valid and relevant given the patient's age and frailty. If the practitioner answers no to this question, the drug should be stopped. However, if the indication appears relevant, the practitioner should then consider if the possible adverse reactions to the medication outweigh the benefits in a patient who is old and frail. If the adverse reactions outweigh the benefits, the drug should be discontinued by way of a taper if necessary. If the practitioner believes the medication continues to provide benefit, the next step would be to determine if there are any side effects from the medication. If the answer is yes, the practitioner should consider switching the medication to another "safer" alternative. However, if the answer is "no," then the practitioner should ask if there is another drug that may be superior to the one in question (i.e., less expensive alternative, more expensive but safer alternative, etc.) If another drug is superior, the practitioner should consider shifting to that drug. Should there be no superior agent, the practitioner should consider if the dose could be reduced and should do so if no significant risk is present. Otherwise, the practitioner should continue with the same dose.

Discuss the following with the patient/guardian

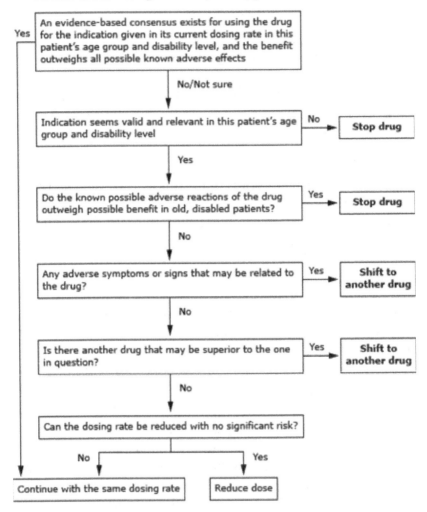

Figure 9-1. The Garfinkel Method[59]

Dr. Garfinkel developed this algorithm by testing it on a cohort of 70 community-dwelling patients. Through the implementation of this algorithm, Dr. Garfinkel was able to discontinue 81 percent of medications he trialed this on. Only 2 percent were restarted, and no significant adverse events were attributable to discontinuation over a 13-month follow-up.[59]

Chapter 10
Summary and Recommendations

Never before have doctors had such an abundance of therapeutic medicinal options. And not surprisingly, the elderly consume more medications than ever before in history. Patients are taking more medications than ever. Both pharmacokinetic and pharmacodynamic changes lead to increased plasma drug concentrations and increased drug sensitivity, and aging influences every aspect of physiologic drug processing. As such, when evaluating older adults, the possibility of an adverse drug event (ADE) should always be considered. Additionally, new symptoms should be considered drug-related until proven otherwise.

Clinicians must be alert to drug-drug interactions, identifying medications that should not be prescribed, or those that should be prescribed with caution, and consider the individual patient.

A step-wise approach to prescribing for older adults should include the following: consider non-pharmacologic alternative strategies; provide a periodic review of current drug therapy; discontinue medications that may no longer be necessary; consider safer alternatives using the appropriate dose; and include those medications that are beneficial to both outcomes and quality of life.

Since the elderly segment is expanding more rapidly than any other cohort of the population, to recognize and prevent problems associated with medications is one of the most critical safety and economic issues facing the healthcare system today. Since this problem demands multidisciplinary involvement, everyone from families to practitioners can play a key role in making a difference.

References

1 US Census Bureau. (2012). Population Division.

2 Hanlon, J.T., Schmader, K.E., et al. (1997). Adverse drug events in high-risk older outpatients. *J Am Geriatr Soc*, 45:945-948.

3 Qiuping, G.U., et al. (September 2010). Prescription drug use continues to increase: *US Prescription Drug Data for 2007-2008*. NCHS Data Brief No. 42.

4 Jackson, M.G., Drechsler-Martell, C.R., Jackson, E.A. (1985). Family practice residents' prescribing patterns. *Drug Intell Clin Pharm*, Mar; 19(3):205-209.

5 Pleym, H., Spigset, O., et al. (2003). Gender differences in drug effects: implications for anesthesiologists. *Acta Anasethsiol Scand*, 47:241-259.

6 Petrone K, Katz P. Approaches to appropriate drug prescribing for the older adult. *Prim Car*. 2005 Sep;32(3):755-775.

7 National Kidney Foundation, 2002. Retrived March 4, 2012, from http://www.kidney.org/professionals/kdoqi/guidelines_ckd/p5_lab_g4.htm.

8 Simon J et al. Interpreting the estimated glomerular filtration rate in primary care: benefits and pitfalls. *Clev Clin J Med*. 2011; 78(3):189-195.

9 Smith GL et al. Renal impairment and outcomes in heart failure: systematic review and meta-analysis. *J Am Coll Cardiol*. 2006; 47: 1987-1996.

10 Smith GL. Serum urea, nitrogen, creatinine, and estimators of renal function. Mortality in older patients with cardiovascular disease. *Arch Intern Med*. 2006; 166: 1134-1142.

11 Adapted from: Pacala JT, Sullivan GM, eds. Geriatrics Review [Syllabus] A Core Curriculum in Geriatric Medicine. 7th ed. New York: *American Geriatrics Society*; 2010.

12 Steinman MA, Landefeld CS, Rosenthal GE, et al. Polypharmacy and prescribing quality in older people. *J Am Geriatr Soc* 2006; 54:1516

13 Hamilton HJ, Gallagher PF, et al. Inappropriate prescribing and adverse drug events in older people. *BMC Geriatrics* 2009; 9:5

14 Bond, CA, Raehl CL, Adverse drug reactions in United States Hospitals. *Pharmacotheraqpy*. 2006;26(5): 601-608

15 Lazarou J et al. *JAMA*. 1998;279(15): 1200-1206

16 Denham MJ. Adverse drug reactions. *Br Med Bull*. 1990;46(1): 53-62.

17 Davies, G., (2011). Polypharmacy and Adverse Drug Reactions (ADR) in the Elderly. Retrieved March 8, 2012, from http://www.docstoc.com/docs/77757229/Poly-pharmacy-and-Adverse-Drug-Reactions-in-the-Elderly.

18 Porter RS, Kaplan JL et al. (2009, Sepetmber). The Merck Manual for Health Care Professionals. Sept 2009. Retrived on March 8, 2012 from http://www.merckmanuals.com/professional/geriatrics.html.

19 Rochon PA, Gurwitz JH. Optimizing drug treatment in elderly people: the prescribing cascade. *BMJ* 1977;315:1097

20 Mosby's Medical Dictionary, 8th edition. 2009

21 2003 Beers Criteria as noted in Poehl, B., Talati, A., Parks, S. (2006). Medication prescribing for older adults. *Ann Long-Term Care.* June; 14(6)33-9.

22 Food and Drug Administration. (2012). *New Molecular Entity Approvals for 2011. U.S.* Retrieved May 2012, from http://www.fda.gov/Drugs/DevelopmentApprovalProcess/DrugInnovation/ucm285554.htm.

23 FDA Approved drugs. (2012). *U.S. Food and Drug Administration.* Retrieved May 2012, from: http://www.centerwatch.com/drug-information/fda-approvals/default.aspx?DrugYear=2-11.

24 Carrillo, J.A., Herraiz, A.G., Ramos, S.I., et al. (2003). Role of the smoking-induced cytochrome P450 (CYP) 1A2 and polymorphic CYP2D6 in steady- state concentration of olanzapine. *J Clin Psychopharmacology*, 23:119-127.

25 Amir, O., Hassan, Y., et al. (2009). Incidence of risk factors for developing hyperkalemia when using ACE inhibitors in cardiovascular diseases. *Pharm World Sci.* June; 31(3):387-93.

26 The American Geriatrics Society. (2012). 2012 Beers Criteria Update Expert Panel. AGS updated Beers Criteria for potentially inappropriate medication use in older adults. *J Am Geriatr Soc.*

27 Wyse, D.G., Waldo, A.L., DiMarco, J.P., et al. (2002). A comparison of rate control and rhythm control in patients with atrial fibrillation. *N Engl J Med*, 347:1825-1833.

28 Carlsson, J., Miketic, S., Windeler, J., et al.(2003). Randomized trial of rate-control versus rhythm-control in persistent atrial fibrillation: the strategies of treatment of atrial fibrillation (STAF) study. *J Am Coll Cardiology*, 41:1690-1696.

29 Ahmed, A. (2007). Digoxin and reduction in mortality and hospitalization in geriatric heart failure: importance of low doses and low serum concentrations. *J Gerontol A Biol Sci Med Sci*, 62(3):323-329.

30 Nifedipine. (1995). Dose-related increase in mortality in patients with coronary heart disease. *Circulation*, 92(5):1326-1331.

31 Juurlink, D.N., Mamdani, M.M., Lee, D.S., et al. (2004). Rates of hyperkalemia after publication of the Randomize Aldactone Evaluation Study. *N Engl J Med*, 351(6):543-551.

32 Fong, T.J., Tulebaev, S.R., et al. (2009). Delirium in elderly adults: diagnosis, prevention and treatment. Nat Rev Neurol, 5(4):210-220.

33 Coupland, C., Dhiman, P., Morriss, R., Arthur, A., Barton, G., and Hippisley-Cox, J. (2001). Antidepressant use and risk of adverse outcomes in older people: population-based cohort study. *BMJ*, 343:d4551.

34 Allain, H., Bentue-Ferrer, D., Polard, E., et al. (2005). Postural instability and consequent falls and hip fractures associated with use of hypnotics in the elderly: a comparative review. *Drugs Aging*, 22(9):749-765.

35 Keston, M., Brocklehurst, J.C. (1974). Flurazepam and meprobamate: a clinical trial. *Age Ageing*. 3(1):54-58.

36 Finkle, W.D., Der, J.S., Greenland, S., et al. (2011). Risk of fractures requiring hospitalization after an initial prescription of zolpidem, alprazolam, lorazepam or diazepam in older adults. *J Am Geriatr Soc*, 599100;1883-1890

37 Cotroneo, A., Gareri, P., Nicoletti, N., et al. (2007). Effectiveness and safety of hypnotic drugs in the treatment of insoeia in over-70-year-old people. *Arch Gerontol Geriatr*, 44(SUPPL 1):121-124.

38 Hulley, S., Grady, D., Bush, T., et al. (1998). Randomized trial of estrogen plus progestin for secondary prevention of coronary heart disease in postmenopausal women. *JAMA*, 280:606-613

39 Writing Group for the Women's Health Initiative Investigators (2002). Risks and benefits of estrogen plus progestin in healthy postmenopausal women: principal results from the Women's Health Initiative randomized controlled trial. JAMA, 288(3):321-333.

40 Hirsch, I.B. (2009). Sliding scale insulin—time to stop sliding. *JAMA*, Jan 14;301(2):213-214.

41 Shorr, R.I., Ray, W.A., Daugherty, J.R., et al. (1996). Individual sulfonylureas and serious hypoglycemia in older people. *J Am Geriatr Soc*, 44(7):751-755.

42 Moertel, C.G., Reitemeier, R.J., Gage, R.P. (1963). A controlled clinical evaluation of anti-emetic drugs. *JAMA*, 186:116-118.

43 Simmons, A., Rouf, E., Whittle ,J. (n.d.). Not your typical pneumonia: a case of exogenous lipoid pneumonia. *J Gen Intern Med.* 22(11):1613-1616.

44 Bateman, D.N., Rawlins, M.D., Simpson, J.M. (1985). Extrapyramidal reactions with metoclopramide. *Br Med J* (Clin Res Ed), 291(6500):930-932.

45 Onder, G., Pellicciotti, F., Gambassi, G., et al. (2004). NSAID-related psychiatric adverse events: who is at risk? *Drugs,* 64(23):2619-2627.

46 Billups, S.J., Delate, T., Hoover, B. (2011). Injury in an elderly population before and after initiating a skeletal muscle relaxant. *Ann Pharmacother*, 45(4):485-491.

47 Gallagher, P., Ryan, C., et al. (2008). Screening tool of older person's prescriptions (STOPP) and screening tool to alert doctors to right treatment (START). Consensus validation. *Int J Clin Pharmacol Ther,* 46:72-83.

48 Feary, J.R., Rodrigues, L.C., et al. (2010). Prevalence of major comorbidities in subjects with COPD and incidence of myocardial infarction and stroke: a comprehensive analysis using data from primary care. *Thorax,* 65:956-962.

49 Lanas ,A., Wu, P., et al. (2001). Low doses of acetylsalicylic acid increase risk of gastrointestinal bleeding in a meta-analysis. *Clin Gastroenterol Hepatol,* 2011;9:762-768.

50 Berger, J.S., Roncaglioni, M.C., et al. (2006). Aspirin for the primary prevention of cardiovascular events in women and men: a sex-specific meta-analysis of randomized controlled trials. *JAMA,* 295(3):306-313.

51 U.S. Preventive Services Task Force. (March 2009). Aspirin for the prevention of cardiovascular disease: recommendation statement. *AHRQ,* Publication No. 09-05129-EF-2,

52 Jacob, S., Spinler, S., (2006). Hyponatremia associated with selective serotonin-reuptake inhibitors in older adults. *Ann Pharmacother,* 40:1618-1622.

53 Organization W. Analgesic Ladder. *World Health Organization;* 1986

54 Mitchell, S.L., Teno, J.M., Kiely, D.K., et al. (2009). The clinical course of advanced dementia. *N Engl J Med,* 361:1529.

55 Hanlon, J.T., Schmader, K.E., Samsa, G.P., et al. (1992). A method for assessing drug therapy appropriateness. *J Clin Eoidermiol,* 45:1045.

56 Steinman, M.A., Landefeld, C.S., Rosenthal, G.E., et al. (2006). Polypharmacy and prescribing quality in older people. *J Am Geriatr Soc,* 54:1516.

57 Appel, L.J., Espeland, M.A., Easter, L., et al. (2001). Effects of reduced sodium intake on hypertension control in older individuals: results from the Trial of Nonpharmacologic Interventions in the Elderly (TONE). *Arch Intern Med,* 161:685.

58 Advancing Adherence & the Science of Pharmacy Care. (June 2011). PQA/URAC Medication Adherence Summit.

59 Garfinkel, D., Mangin, D. (2010). Feasibility study of a systematic approach for discontinuation of multiple medications in older adults: Addressing polypharmacy. *Arch Intern Med,* 170:1648.

Figure & Table Index